JOURNALING CANCER
IN WORDS AND IMAGES

Art Therapy Conference
Savannah —
Harriet Wadeson presentation

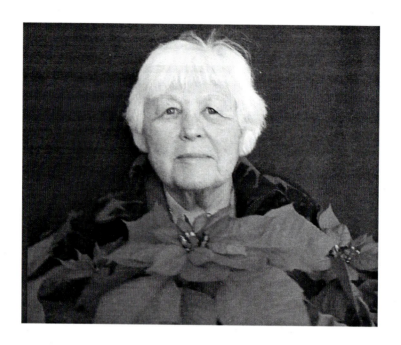

ABOUT THE AUTHOR/ARTIST

Harriet Claire Wadeson is a pioneer in art therapy, beginning her career in 1961 at the National Institutes of Health (NIH), where she worked for thirteen years. She directed the Art Therapy Graduate Program at the University of Houston for two years and at the University of Illinois at Chicago for twenty-three years, including its Annual Summer Institute at Lake Geneva, WI, which she directed for twenty years. She has published seven books in art therapy, approximately seventy papers in refereed journals, and numerous chapters in art therapy and psychology textbooks. Her awards include the Benjamin Rush Bronze Medal Award from the American Psychiatric Association for her scientific exhibit *Portraits of Suicide;* First Prize for research from the American Art Therapy Association, First Prize for art from the Smithsonian Institute, Washington, DC; a Resolution of Commendation from the Illinois Legislature; a Distinguished Faculty Award from Northwestern University; and Honorary Life Membership (HLM) from the American Art Therapy Association, art therapy's highest honor. She has served on the Executive Board of that organization as well as serving as its research chair, publications chair, honors chair, ethics chair, newsletter editor, and associate editor of its journal *Art Therapy*. She has been an international guest lecturer, faculty, and workshop leader in fourteen countries, and has led professional delegations to China, Java, Bali, and Sweden. She maintained a private therapy, art therapy, and professional supervision practice for many years. Currently she directs the Art Therapy Certificate Program at Northwestern University, continues her painting, and is working on three novels.

JOURNALING CANCER IN WORDS AND IMAGES

Caught in the Clutch of the Crab

By

HARRIET CLAIRE WADESON, Ph.D., LCSW, ATR-BC, HLM

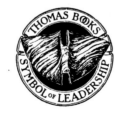

CHARLES C THOMAS • PUBLISHER, LTD.
Springfield • Illinois • U.S.A.

Published and Distributed Throughout the World by

CHARLES C THOMAS • PUBLISHER, LTD.
2600 South First Street
Springfield, Illinois 62704

© 2011 by CHARLES C THOMAS • PUBLISHER, LTD.

ISBN 978-0-398-08672-5 (paper)
ISBN 978-0-398-08673-2 (ebook)

Library of Congress Catalog Card Number: 2011015037

With THOMAS BOOKS *careful attention is given to all details of manufacturing
and design. It is the Publisher's desire to present books that are satisfactory as to their
physical qualities and artistic possibilities and appropriate for their particular use.*
THOMAS BOOKS *will be true to those laws of quality that assure a good name
and good will.*

Printed in the United States of America
MM-R-3

Library of Congress Cataloging-in-Publication Data

Wadeson, Harriet, 1931–
Journaling cancer in words and images : caught in the clutch of the
crab / by Harriet Claire Wadeson.
 p. cm.
Includes bibliographical references.
ISBN 978-0-398-08672-5 (pbk.) -- ISBN 978-0-398-08673-2 (ebook)
1. Wadeson, Harriet, 1931–Health. 2. Cancer–Patients–United States–
Biography. 3. Psychotherapists–United States–Biography. I. Title.

RC265.6.W33W33 2011
362.196'9940092–dc23

2011015037

This work is dedicated to Neena Schwartz,
who stayed steadfastly by my side on this difficult journey.
Neither words nor pictures can convey the significance
of having a loving companion when facing the
terrors from the clutch of the crab.

ACKNOWLEDGMENTS

My gratitude goes to my many caregivers who helped to save my life, particularly my oncologist Dr. Gustavo Rodriguez, for being a warm and caring physician, even though I may have made him impatient with my repeated questions. My appreciation goes as well to the countless researchers and practitioners, people I do not know, who have worked tirelessly to develop treatments for cancer. I'd like to acknowledge also those sensitive individuals who recognize the extensive emotional needs of cancer patients and have established programs and services to meet such needs. It is so very important to know that you are not alone in confronting the whirlwind of emotions cancer generates.

Many people have been helpful to me in creating this book, both in their encouragement and in their reading of the manuscript. My Portia Group of exceptional women scholars, writers, and artists was the first to hear portions of the journal with accompanying pictures. Their heartfelt enthusiasm for the work prompted me to move toward publication. My friend Sue Roupp, writer, editor, writing teacher, actor, and TV moderator, was the first to read the full manuscript. Her encouragement was exuberant, and her suggestions very useful. Another good friend, Margherita Andreotti, writer, editor, and art historian, read this manuscript with great thoughtfulness and viewed the artwork with particular sensitivity to its importance. I am appreciative of her many kindnesses during my illness in addition to her cogent suggestions for this book. Maxine Borowsky Junge, dear friend and colleague, read the book as soon as I sent it to her and replied immediately with very helpful suggestions. I am especially appreciative of her perspective as a sister art therapist whose views I have respected over our many years helping to grow this profession and through our various collaborations as art therapy authors and editors. In spite of being so close to the experience recounted, Neena Schwartz was able to step back and view the writing from the perspective of an academic, offering valuable suggestions about its construction and tolerating my descriptions of our interactions. My gratitude goes to Michael Payne Thomas, President of Charles C Thomas Publisher, for his support of this somewhat unusual book and for his generous offer to purchase equipment to produce the accompanying CD.

And finally, many thanks to all those who kept me in their thoughts and prayers throughout my siege of cancer treatment. The significance of such support is beyond description.

CONTENTS

Page

Chapter

JOURNALING CANCER
IN WORDS AND IMAGES

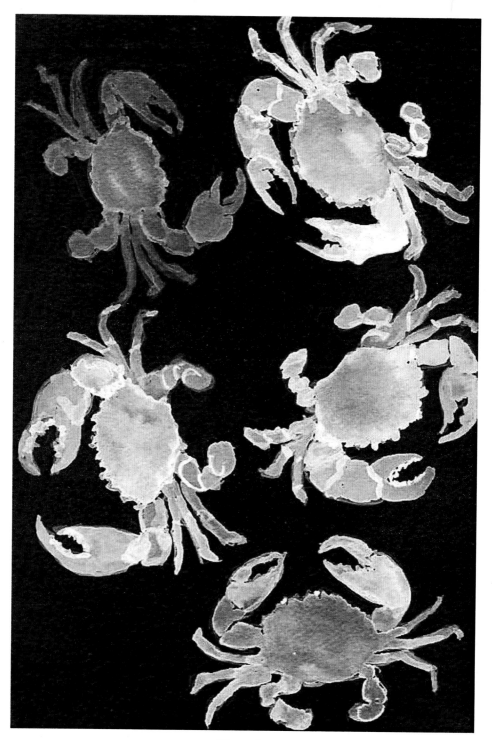

Figure 1.

1

INTRODUCTION

The American Cancer Society reports that cancer is the second leading cause of death in the United States. The disease is epidemic. In this country, 41 percent of the population, half of all men and more than one third of all women, will have cancer during their lifetimes. Probably all of us will have to deal with cancer, either our own or in a loved one, at some time in our lives. Even without this dismal statistic, many of us harbor a horror of cancer. More than other prevalent illnesses, such as heart disease and stroke, cancer conjures up fears of suffering, helpless debilitation, and death.

This is a book I never intended to write. My seven other books are about art therapy, a field in which I have worked for almost fifty years. I began at a time when most people had never heard of art therapy and very little was written about it. Because I entered the profession in its infancy, I am considered something of an art therapy pioneer. Although my books include my own reactions to my clients and to the work, I never intended to write a book in which I was the single case example, but then, I never expected to be diagnosed with cancer.

My own reaction was that I needed to tell my story. Because I am an art therapist, I needed to tell it in images as well as in words. This book is the result. It is very intimate. A problem in publishing any memoir is the concern about what is better left unsaid, particularly publicly unsaid. Obviously, that includes what might be hurtful to others. In my case, it also comprises some symptoms that were pretty disgusting. Should good taste dictate their omission? My conflict has been that I have wanted this book to be completely open and honest, the full experience of my illness. So in addition to awful side effects, sometimes inadequate or rough treatment, and insensitive remarks from friends, I have also included moments that are frankly embarrassing, when I have lost my temper or harbored resentful feelings towards others. I imagine my friends, colleagues, and students reading these passages and worry about whether they will ever respect me again. My hope is that my all-too-human frailties will warrant some forgiveness, if not identification.

Although I wrote the journal and created the artwork only for myself, toward the end of my treatment I began to think that this combination of words and images might be meaningful to others. Dealing with serious illness and the threat of death is so much a part of the human experience that it seemed to me that using the combination of writing and art in traversing the treacherous terrain of Cancer Land could be of interest to others.

More specifically, I hope that the book will be meaningful to those on this journey and helpful to the people who care for them in increasing their understanding and in enabling them to provide treatment with greater sensitivity. For myself, the publication of this work is a sort of validation, a need to have something good come from the fear and suffering cancer brings.

The book is divided into five sections: (1) A brief passage about *Creative Expression;* (2) *In the Clutch of the Crab,* the daily journal I kept along with digressions into issues that concerned me; (3) *Surviving,* discussions of follow-up experience in the year after treatment and further significant issues; (4) *Cancer Land,* the altered book I created of paintings and collages of my treatment, accompanied by a CD of the images in full color (located at the back of the book); (5) a discussion of *Writing and Making Art* about my cancer journey with a comparison of these two modes of expression, in which my experience of each was vastly different from the other.

My preference would be to include color reproductions of the artwork in the text of the written journal, but that would make this book far too expensive. So the pictures that accompany the written experience are shown in black and white in the journal text but may be seen in color on the CD. Most are from the altered book I made. I discussed the artwork only minimally as I wrote the journal, but it is reviewed in Section 5, *Cancer Land,* which is about the altered book. I am very happy to include a CD so that all the pictures can be viewed in full color. They are a particularly important component of this work. I hope that readers will view the CD as they are reading the *Cancer Land, An Altered Book* section, rather than interrupting reading the written journal to look at the pictures in color.

Although there is some inevitable repetition in this twice-told tale, I believe the words and the images tell their stories in different ways and ultimately enhance one another to give a full picture of life in Cancer Land. ✳ Key

Because this book is such a personal account of one of the most ✳ threatening experiences of my life, I feel very vulnerable in sending it out into the world to be viewed not only by friends and colleagues, but also by people I don't even know. I have valued responses to my other books, so I am especially eager for the personal responses that I hope the personal nature of this book will prompt. hope/Belief.

I believe that one day cancer treatment will be more specific to target only cancer cells, rather than the current sledgehammer approach that destroys so many other cells and disrupts bodily processes. That is a goal of current research, but I doubt that I will live long enough to see cancer treatment become more humane as a result.

Color is important to her...

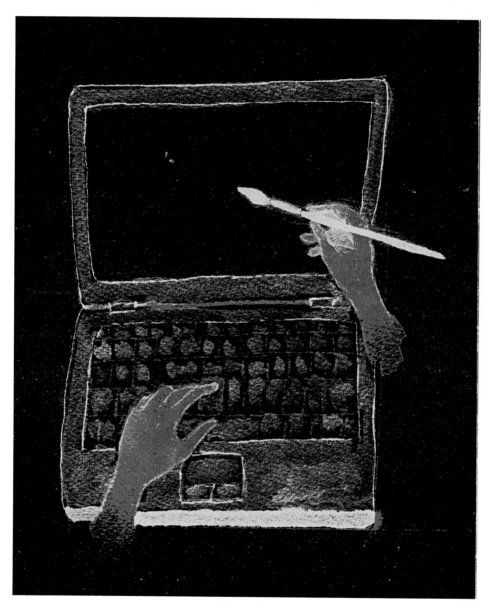

Figure 2.

2

CREATIVE EXPRESSION

"C"

Cancer imposed its own special kind of helplessness as I was cut open and parts were either removed or irradiated and blasted with chemicals that destroyed cells and interfered with my physiological functioning. Others have turned to a number of outlets under this kind of duress–religion, meditation, music–I don't know what else. For me, I needed to *do* something, to be active to oppose my resignation to the tortures imposed upon me. I needed to assert my personhood as I passively underwent frightening, debilitating, and humiliating procedures. Writing and making art were my saviors in times of trouble or pain in the past, so it was only natural for me to turn to them to help me through the cancer challenge to my life.

Before + during + after

I began a journal the day I was diagnosed. I am not sure what I had in mind, but I think it was to anchor myself during the heavy buffeting for which I knew I was headed. What I have found is that had I not written about it, I would have forgotten much of what I experienced. So, unintentionally, the journal has been a kind of record keeping as well.

I took my paints with me to the hospital when I had surgery, my first treatment shortly after I was diagnosed, but I was unable to use them the few days I was there. I started painting soon after coming home, however, beginning with plants and flowers friends brought. My first cancer picture was of my hand taped with the tube infusing me with chemicals and the pole with the beeping chemo machine behind it that I painted in my first chemotherapy session. There were other paintings, but they did not get organized until I attended an altered book workshop. Creating a book was a powerful impetus to tell my story in images.

As far as I know, no one has combined writing and art in this way to publish the experience of cancer. The closest work I know is the art and writing of artist Hollis Sigler, who created a *Breast Cancer Journal* in paintings (1999). She wrote on the paintings and about the artwork, but her subject was her effort to publicize the prevalence of breast cancer at a time when its epidemic proportion was unrecognized.

I was faithful to both endeavors, writing in my journal and tracing my cancer journey in images, throughout my treatment. I found these two modalities to be very different experiences, not only in how I was expressing myself, but also in what I was expressing, which I discuss at the end of this book. In telling my story in these two different modes of expression simultaneously, I found that each enhanced the other.

The art I created was relatively quick, made with simple materials. Most of the time I was working on it, I was too depleted for more extended projects. The same is true of the writing. So much of the material is raw—spontaneous journal entries and pictures made when I was feeling very ill. In a way, however, these spontaneous expressions of what was happening to me and my resultant feelings are perhaps more genuine than refined writing and art making would be.

I recall a visit to the Guggenheim Museum when I was a young woman to see an exhibit of famous artists' sketchbooks. I was amazed. Max Beckman did not seem to know how to draw hands! The purpose of this exhibit was to display preparatory work, not what was created to be shown. I hope the work presented here can be received with the same understanding of the circumstances of its creation and not be judged on aesthetic merit but rather as expressions of my day to day journey through Cancer Land.

I think creative expression is very important for those living in dread of a possibly fatal illness and undergoing harsh, debilitating medical treatment. Cancer is life sucking. It is easy to become your cancer with all the medical appointments and treatment side effects that take over your life. Cancer can suck out all other life you have.

In *The Emperor of All Maladies,* an amazing book recounting the history of cancer discoveries and treatment, Siddhartha Mukherjee (2010) describes cancer's takeover more eloquently than I have. He compares life with cancer to the personal "annihilation" in a concentration camp's "erasure of the future. . . . Cancer is not a concentration camp, but it shares the quality of annihilation: it negates the possibility of life outside and beyond itself; it subsumes all living. The daily life of a patient becomes so intensely preoccupied with his or her illness that the world fades away. Every last morsel of energy is spent tending the disease."

Writing and painting, however, even if about the pain in your current reality, lifts you beyond that reality into a world of your own creation. There is a strange paradox here. Although the focus is on what may be suffering, perhaps even the reliving of an excruciating experience, that focus is enveloped by another focus, which is the creative experience itself. While writing about nausea from chemotherapy, for example, I was also selecting the best words to describe it. Sometimes I could find satisfaction and even pleasure in perhaps pairing just the right words. This same sort of creative involvement was even more intense in making art. Instead of words, I would be selecting and composing images and enjoying the sensual pleasures of manipulating materials with the stroke of a paintbrush or applying glossy satin ribbons. So, although writing or painting about nausea, I was enjoying my own creative activity. Afterwards, I would look at my creation and smile. Yes, I would think, that is what it is like.

What's more, creative self-expression can affirm your own special personhood, what in you is strong and unique. You are not simply a cipher in an unending march of patients into the operating room, the radiology department, the chemotherapy suite. You are expressing your own individual response to the tsunami that has wrecked your life and the flood that is drowning so much of it.

I have found creative self-expression to be a bridge as well, reaching across the abyss of cancer to others so they can know what it is like to live in the clutch of the crab. I recall a young woman who approached me after I had presented the art from *Cancer Land,* my altered book, at an art therapy professional conference. Her mother had had cancer. "I never knew what chemo was like for her before," she told me.

I feel very fortunate that both writing and making art were already old friends when the tsunami hit. I did not have to look for them, they were already by my side to help keep me afloat through the ebbs and flows of the strong tides of cancer that washed over me.

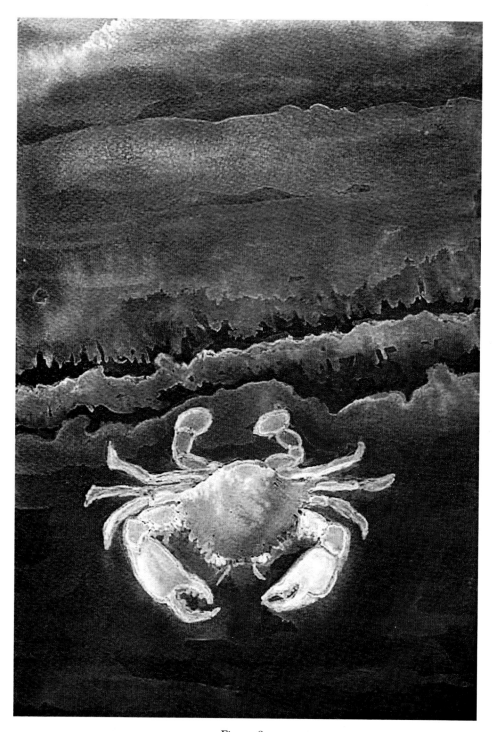

Figure 3.

3

IN THE CLUTCH OF THE CRAB:
A CANCER JOURNAL

CANCER THE CRAB

*C*ancer, the astrological crab, governs female reproductive organs, the stomach, and digestion. Cancer, the disease, however, can affect many other
parts of the body as well. This crab scuttles all over the world, clutching many
of us in its claws.

*When Hippocrates, considered the father of medicine, saw the cut surface of
a breast cancer, he described it as a crab,* carcinos *in Greek, because it looked
like that creature with its legs stretching outwards. He coined the word* carcinoma, *meaning crab swelling. The Roman physician Celsus translated it into
the Latin* cancer, *which means gangrene as well.*

APRIL 14

"At age seventy-eight, you don't need anymore Pap tests," Dr.
Stewart says, turning to me from her computer. She is a slight woman
with a warm smile, who always greets me with a handshake. "If the last
three have been good, you don't need anymore."

"When was my last one?"

She returns to the computer, which she spends more time examining than me, as though my truth is contained in that machine, rather
than in my body. "Three years ago," the computer tells her.

"I'm sure I've had one more recently."

"Strange," she clicks the computer some more, "your records show
an appointment last year, but no results."

I've never been concerned about my Pap tests. They're just routine, so I probably didn't even notice that I never got a result.

"In that case, why don't you do one last one," I suggest.

I climb up on the table and lie back. She palpates my abdomen and does a breast exam. I put my feet in the humiliating stirrups and scoot my butt down to the end of the table. The speculum is cold and hard. Then the swab pokes my cervix. Hooray for the last time.

APRIL 17

Stewart calls. The Pap test shows atypical glandular cells. She explains that they are normal in menstruating women, but abnormal postmenopause.

"What could they indicate?"

"Cancer." The first mention of that word.

"Anything else?"

"Precancer. Or sometimes there is no explanation."

What is my uterus up to? Does she think she's still young, that her ovaries can still produce eggs? Maybe she is trying to grow another baby. Or perhaps something else is growing there, not birth but death. I'm not worried though. I figure I am in the "no explanation" category. The body often defies medical testing.

Stewart is a very thorough primary physician who refers to specialists readily to make sure all bases are covered. Since she is an internist, she wants me to see a gynecologist to determine if I need a biopsy. She gives me the names of three women who are a part of the same North Shore Health System as she is, a large organization comprising several hospitals and office buildings in the suburbs north of metropolitan Chicago. The best thing about the system is the internet (even Stewart's computer). My doctors can access all of my records with a couple of clicks, and we can communicate with each other through their e-mail system.

I call and make an appointment with the doctor with the earliest opening.

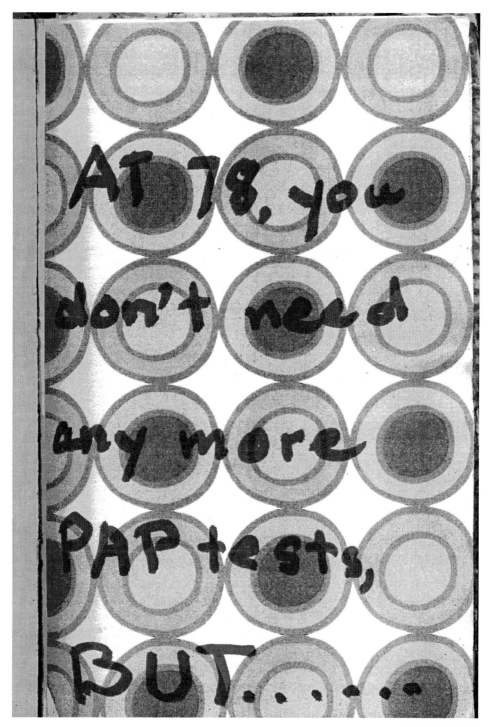

Figure 4. Internist's announcement.

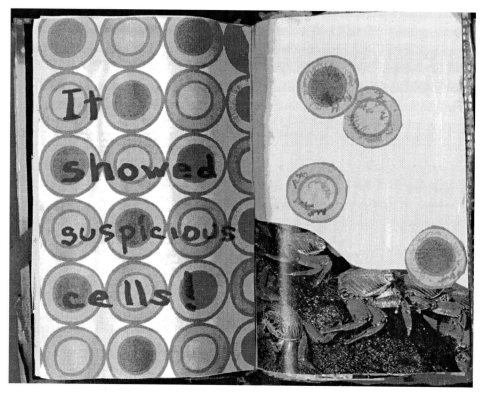

Figure 5. Pap test results.

APRIL 30

Dr. Swenson is a pretty blond young woman in a spacious new office building with blond furniture. Because she looks so young, I ask her how long she has been with North Shore, and she gives me her history—something like eight years, going back to training at Hopkins. It must be a sign of old age that everyone looks young enough to be my grandchild. A couple of months ago, I had a stress test at this same facility, and the cardiologist, who told me that my heart was stronger than his, looked about fourteen years old.

There is no question about doing a biopsy of the endometrium, so I'm in the stirrups—back in the saddle again. Swenson rigs up a light and a screen so I can view the proceedings inside me, but I turn away, too chicken to watch.

MAY 7

Swenson calls with the biopsy results: more glandular cells in the uterus, but the cervix looks fine. It could be pre-cancer, but I will need a D&C [dilatation and curettage] for a complete diagnosis. The schedule for the outpatient surgery OR [operating room] at Evanston Hospital is crowded. Her office can't find a slot for me until May 22, two weeks later.

DRUNK DRIVER, MAY 8

Life careens out of control, as does cancer and the drunk driver who smashes into my car. At midnight, my partner Neena and I are asleep when the phone rings. It's Connie, our next-door neighbor, and in my stupor I think she says she's been hit by a car. I ask her if she is okay and where she is.

"I'm in my house. A car has smashed into your car."

I wake Neena, throw a jacket on over my nightgown, and rush outside. Police lights are flashing, neighbors have congregated, and my green Subaru Forester is on the sidewalk, its rear smashed into the front seat. The lawn is splattered with shattered glass. I try to think clearly enough to take essentials out of the car, like the registration card, before a tow truck hauls it away. The rear of Neena's Prius, which was parked in front of mine, is wrecked too, but not as bad. Hers is drivable, so it remains. The policeman points out that there are no skid marks, the guy never even tried to stop. He is sitting in an ambulance across the street, having been nabbed by the cop after running through Connie's yard to the back alley. Not a kid, a fifty-five-year-old man who lives a few blocks away. So much for our nice suburban neighbors.

Here I am, facing a possible serious diagnosis and needing a car. I rent one and go car shopping. I make a decision quickly instead of doing my usual obsessive research. Another Forester, this time red.

Neena and I go to car hell, the junkyard where my car was towed, so I can get more stuff out of the wreck. It's a car graveyard with all of them piled up against one another. Several have to be moved by forklift for me to get to mine.

I liked my old car. The new SUVs are too big, but a car is such a small concern when your body may be in jeopardy.

DOOR COUNTY, MAY 15–20

Neena owns a cottage in the woods on a bluff in Door County, WI, overlooking Ellison Bay, which is an offshoot of Green Bay, which is a large offshoot of Lake Michigan. I love it there, and now that both of us are retired from academia, we can go there whenever we want. Spring is very special in Door County. We have a week before the D&C. After driving the 250 miles north along Lake Michigan, I feel as though I've gone back in time. Up north, it is an earlier spring than at home, with leaves a delicate new green, wild flowers sprinkled throughout the still partially bare woods, and a chorus of peepers singing nightly in the marshes by Neena's house. There are basses and sopra-

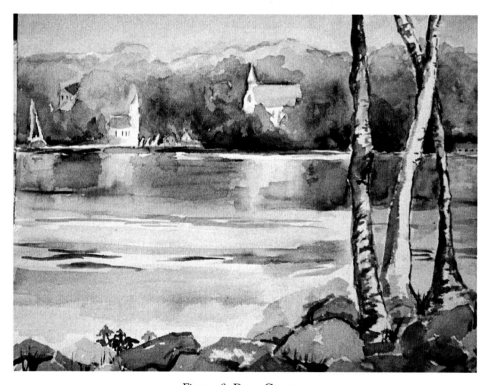

Figure 6. Door County.

nos and everything in between. We walk through woods carpeted with white trillium, and I take a longer walk by myself on the Lynd trail by Lake Michigan that skirts layered outcroppings of moss-covered limestone. I need Door County right now. Going back in time isn't bad either.

All the sheets have gotten musty, so I pack them to take home to launder, confident that I will be returning in a month for the summer.

CANCER, DAY 1, MAY 27

I have the D&C on Friday, May 22, in outpatient surgery, barely an event at all, and make an appointment to get the results in a week. Swenson's office calls on Tuesday, four days later, to say she is going out of town so I should come in for my follow-up appointment the next day. Strange. . . . Then in the evening someone else from her office calls saying the same thing, that she needs to reschedule me for tomorrow. I ask if she is going out of town.

"Not that I know of." The tip-off.

May 27: Neena and I wait an hour and a half in a busy waiting room filled with pregnant women and little kids in a different building and neighborhood from the quiet, serene offices where I'd seen Swenson before. I doze and think about how I can live with cancer. I'm glad I've done most of the writing on my current art therapy book so I won't have pressure from my publisher's deadline of September 1. I'll just do what I want—painting and writing fiction.

Eventually, we are ushered in to the inner sanctum. I suppose it is an examining room, but I don't remember it at all, except that it is small and closed in. We are seated, Neena to my right, but I really don't recall her presence either. I don't remember whether Swenson comes in after us or if she is there already. I tunnel vision her face and see nothing else. She is sitting opposite me, her face close to mine. She looks older, troubled by strain and pain. She apologizes for the "white lie," saying she thought I would want to know right away.

"It's cancer." Those life-changing words.

Swenson says she's surprised. Not the usual kind of uterine cancer. "Serous papillary carcinoma, high grade." I'm used to getting high grades, but this kind sounds ominous. She says I'll have to have a hysterectomy and hands me a sheaf of papers with information on three gynecological oncologists.

"We are lucky to have found it," she adds. A Pap test is designed to discover cervical cancer, but my cervix looks fine.

Is this the first day of my cancer? Of course not. I've been feeling well, unaware of the time bomb ticking deep within me. My insides will be ripped out. At least my uterus and ovaries are not parts of myself I will miss, and it's not as though I have been invaded. Cancer is my own body destroying itself.

My first thoughts stream to my children. How will I tell them? Eric, who lives near San Francisco, is the first to call. I tell him I will have to have a hysterectomy. He asks questions. I answer them. The other kids call from Virginia (I have no family here in the Midwest). They all respond like themselves. Eric is matter-of-fact and tries to be supportive. Lisa is sentimental and loving. Keith tries to put a good face on it. He's going to look up information on the Internet. I tell him I don't want to hear about it.

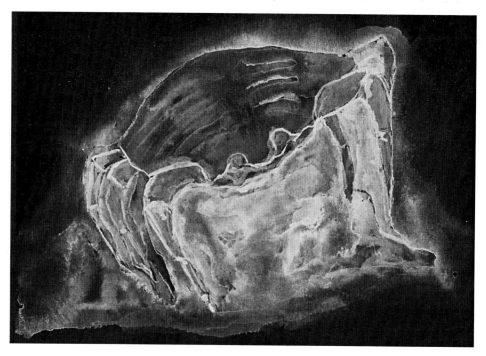

Figure 7. Cancer.

In the evening, I try to explain my life view to Neena, how for years I have lived in awe, each leaf, each blade of grass, a miracle. That I am alive is amazing to me. Of all the millions of possibilities, a particular sperm mated with a particular ovum to become me. Although almost impossible for me to imagine, of course I will die. I just haven't known when or how. I'd always thought I would live into my nineties like my parents.

I digress. I am trying to say that my life is infinitesimally small in the vast universe of space and time. I'm trying to say that in my seventy-eight years I've done most of what I've wanted to do. I'm grateful to Neena and my children, who are all being very loving. Eric's kids, Michaela and Amanda, teen-agers, call too.

But I feel fine! An early symptom of uterine cancer is bleeding. I don't even have that.

CANCER, DAY 2, MAY 28

My life is in the tentacles of the crab. Sometimes I feel sort of cosmic about it all and view it from afar. Other times I dread the medical torture that lies ahead. Sometimes I just go about my business, like working on my art therapy book today. I've decided to live my life, going to a concert tonight and to a play tomorrow night. At least until I see the oncologist June 2.

Neena looks up my diagnosis. She is a famous reproductive biologist. When I take her with me to new medical appointments, the doctors invariably say, "Professor Schwartz, I was in your Northwestern Medical School physiology class." I get good treatment that way. They want to impress their old prof.

Neena discovers that "high grade" means a very aggressive form of cancer. That implodes. I'm in for a rough ride. Is this my last spring? I feel melodramatic when I ask such a question. I don't look up the diagnosis myself. I'm too frightened of what I will find.

CANCER, DAY 4, MAY 30

I am living in dread, seeing myself inserted into the medical machine and ground up. I feel good now but know I'll feel awful after the surgery and wonder if I will ever feel good again. Maybe these are my last days worth living.

Cancer Land is the place from which you never return. It is a place of extreme vulnerability, dread, and the fear that your cancer can always return. It is a place of pain and medical torture, a place of fatigue, weakness, and feeling sick. I have been banished from the relatively carefree place where I used to live. Those who live there still wander in and out of my life. They can see the pain and weariness in my face, but they do not live where I do. There is a glass divide between us. We travel different roads.

I'm not miserable enough–yesterday I fell in the backyard. I stepped into a hole I didn't know was there–a metaphor maybe? The pain in my knee is no metaphor though.

I went to the Friday afternoon writing group anyway and related to the others the way I usually do. No one would know that I can't stop thinking about the cancer. Today I go to the Saturday Farmers Market. It helps to stay active. I plant flowers in the large pots on the deck and the window boxes in front so I'll have them to enjoy after the surgery. I wash the bedroom windows.

Neena is being very sweet to me. We're gentle with each other, the way we should be all the time. Love has been what I've wanted most in my life. How sad that it has taken a fatal disease. . . .

I am carrying horrible images in my head–Susan Sontag on her deathbed photographed by Annie Leibovitz. How could she do that to her partner? Sontag was a proud and powerful woman. I think she would have been pissed to have the world see her so helpless. Recently I read that she died from the blood cancer that was caused by the chemotherapy used to treat her breast cancer.

Eric calls to say that Roy, a childhood friend now an internist, says that if the cancer hasn't spread, treatment should be a snap. That's an idea I want to hold.

DAY 5, MAY 31

I go to a reception on the patio at Three Crowns Retirement Center to celebrate the mural some of us from the Illinois Art Therapy Association painted for them. Mary Frances, a resident, comments on

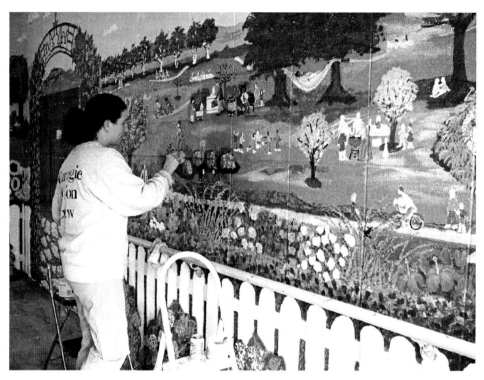

Figure 8. Robinlee painting a mural for Three Crowns.

my beautiful hair, and a week ago a stranger sitting behind me at some event tapped my shoulder to tell me what beautiful hair I have. Most grandmas have short hair and many color it. Mine is shining white, long and thick. I may lose it all.

Robinlee, who has headed up the mural project, hugs me goodbye, saying she'll see me next in Sweden. I am supposed to leave in five days, first to teach art therapy there, as I do every year, then to lead a delegation I organized to make art and celebrate the summer solstice in the beautiful Swedish countryside. I've been planning this trip for a year.

The air is different in rural Sweden, making the colors more vivid. In the small town of Brevens Bruk, where I teach, a bygone monarch ordained that all the stucco buildings had to be painted a creamy golden color, and they are offset by the redwood stain of the wooden buildings. To these hues are added the sparkling blue of the several lakes nearby and the whites and pinks of the profusion of flowers fed by the many hours of sunlight that make the June days extend until midnight. The evenings are especially delicious, stretching the daylight into long liquid hours of softening colors for walks into town down the road arched with trees. I teach in an old schoolhouse with high ceilings that my hosts, Lena and Kenneth, have transformed into an artist's paradise with wonderful studio space set amidst fields and woods. Robin-lee will be one of the art therapists going as part of the delegation. I don't tell her I might not make it.

I e-mail my brother Sonny, saying that he's my poster boy for fighting cancer (fourteen years!). His is renal, a particularly lethal form of cancer. He was doing well for six years following the removal of his kidney, then the cancer returned to other parts of his body. He has had various surgeries, including one in which his heart stopped twice, and the gamma knife, for which his head had to be bolted down while lesions in his brain were irradiated. He tells me that only 6 percent with kidney cancer live ten years, so he considers himself "off the charts." Throughout these fourteen years, he has remained optimistic and cheerful. I say I'll keep the example of his positive attitude in mind as I wage my own battle. I think of how hard it would be for my parents to have both their children suffering from cancer. They lived into their nineties, untouched by it. In spite of Sonny's positive example, I can't stop the images of others I've seen die of cancer–Tory, Marjorie, Mema, Adrienne, Marcia.

JUNE 1

In the morning I go to a party at Jacqui's given by my daily Aqua Fitness group, or "Splashers," as we call ourselves. I haven't gone to the swimming pool since my diagnosis. I try to be present, but it's difficult. I tell my diagnosis to Jacqui and Claire S., and they seem moved. I tell Mary B. too, our unofficial scribe, so she can let the others know why I'll be away for a while. I've decided to get as much support as I can.

In the evening I go to our annual Portia dinner at Lupita's Mexican restaurant. Portia is a group of women scholars, writers, artists, and musicians who meet monthly to present our works in progress to one another. There's much laughter at the table. I wait until the end then drop my news and ask for their support. I'm choked up. They are wonderfully forthcoming.

My usual approach to making choices is to research the possibilities, whether it is a vacation hotel, a new car, or vitamin supplements. I ask my friends, I look on the Web, I read books. In choosing cancer treatment, a much more weighty decision than any of the others, I do not want to run around searching frantically. I do not want to be faced with options. I do not want to look up my specific cancer, serous papillary carcinoma, and read about its horrors.

So, I simply call the number Swenson gave me for a gynecological oncology practice at Evanston Hospital. I do make one choice, however. Of the three oncologists she recommended, I try for the female, but she is about to leave town for six months. So I go with the first doctor available, Gustavo Rodriguez. Neena has worked with the folks at Northwestern University Hospital, and she asks their head of gynecology about him as well as Teresa, a former student who has worked with Rodriguez. They both have good things to say. The Northwestern gynecology head says they would be glad to treat me there, but I'd have to travel downtown each time, and Evanston Hospital is only a few blocks away. I go for convenience. I seem to be trying not to make a big deal of this. Am I crazy?

GUSTAVO RODRIGUEZ, JUNE 2

Gus Rodriguez is a pleasant man with a ready smile. I like him. He doesn't hurry me. He gives me lots of information about different treatments, depending on what he finds inside. If the cancer was confined to the polyp Swenson removed, I won't need more treatment after the surgery. Otherwise, there's chemotherapy and radiation. Before the surgery I'll have to have a CAT [computerized axial tomography] scan to see if it has spread. If it has, then surgery is optional—locking the barn door after the horse has escaped—to prevent pain. That sounds so ominous, I immediately banish it from my consciousness. What comes next isn't any better. Mine is the kind of cancer in which a cell can break off at any time, hit the bloodstream, and relocate. Terrifying. I consider asking if there is a possibility that the lab could have made a mistake, mixed up my results with someone else's, but I don't. Maybe every cancer patient wants to believe that some horrible mistake has been made, that it's someone else's cancerous cells.

Rodriguez is gentle in the exam, even though he is poking around inside me. He apologizes, which seems very sensitive. His nurse Ann is chirpy but sweet. She looks about thirteen.

Should I go to Sweden and have the surgery when I return? Maybe they won't even be able to schedule the OR right away. And Rodriguez will be going on vacation soon. I may have to wait until he returns. It's Tuesday. Rodriguez says there may be an opening Friday because a woman with ovarian cancer is not sure whether she wants the surgery scheduled for her then or not. Ann calls her. She doesn't want it. I tell her to schedule me. How would I enjoy Sweden anyway with cancer treatment hanging in my consciousness, and I don't think "high grade" should be delayed. Bite the bullet. Better not to have too much time to obsess about it.

JUNE 3

I go to my last painting class, the last chance to work in oils from the model. I tell Janis, the teacher, that I am about to have cancer surgery. She says I am courageous to come to class.

I have the CAT scan in the afternoon. I had to drink a barium dye "smoothie" last night and some bitter stuff with iodine in it this morning to light up my insides. As I lie on the table I am injected with more dye that not only lights me within, it heats me up as well. The stuff I drank is supposed to shine on my colon, and the other dye is for visualizing everything else. The table slides me in and out of the ring of the cathode ray machine with an inner ring that whirls around ominously when it's shooting. Looming over me on the machine, a little yellow smiley face in profile lights up with puffed out cheeks, and a voice booms, "Hold your breath," as I slide out. The table stops and a green smiling opened-mouth face lights up as the voice commands, "breathe." I go in and out a number of times to get my pelvis, abdomen, and chest shot. It doesn't take long, and other than the hot dye, there are no physical sensations. But I don't think I've known such terror over a stretch of time, as this machine runs its seek-the-tumor mis-

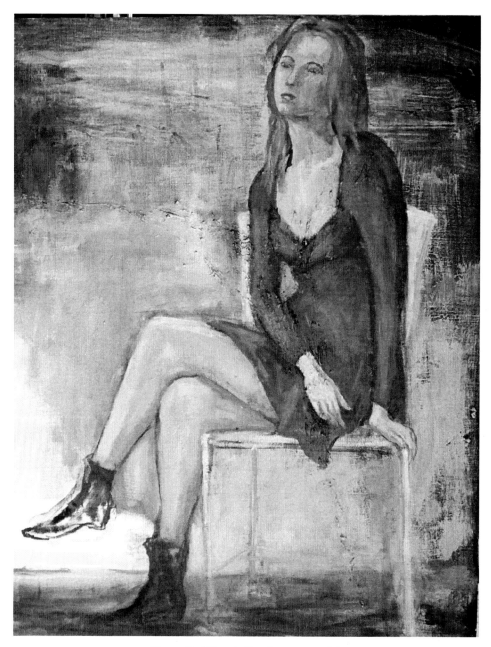

Figure 9. Oil painting from a model.

sion. My back aches horribly with all the tension from the fear that the cancer has spread. I dream about it.

DAY BEFORE SURGERY, JUNE 4

Neena and I wait forty-five minutes to see Rodriguez, who will give me the CAT scan results. Sitting in the dimly lit waiting room, I make the decision to forego surgery if the cancer has spread and try to enjoy what good days I have left and then end it. The terror of spread is overwhelming; I can think of nothing else. When Rodriguez tells me there is no evidence of spread, that the CAT scan shows no changes since a year ago (when I had to have one for a hernia), not even enlarged lymph nodes, I am ecstatic. I tell him I want to kiss him. He looks embarrassed and says he's just the messenger. I blow him a kiss. Here I am, about to have abdominal surgery for cancer, and I am actually happy. I just keep thinking it was a cancerous polyp, nothing more.

I ask Ann how long she has been doing this work because she looks so young. About a year, she says. She adds that she definitely wants to stay in oncology. I can't imagine why anyone would want work with people in torment and terror.

Neena and I have dinner (last supper?) at an Indian restaurant we frequent. It is very good, although I still can eat only less than half. (I've had no appetite since the diagnosis.) We watch a movie on TV, and I am even able to sleep the night before surgery.

SURGERY, JUNE 5

Lying on the gurney curtained off from the other "pre-ops" in the holding room, I tell Rodriguez that many people are sending him their blessings. He says that he prays too. I feel very supported. I e-mailed the art therapy e-group, my daily aqua group, the novel writing group, Portia, and various others in a wise decision to reach out for support. I am amazed at how many contacted me, some I don't even know who have heard me speak or have read my books. Their messages are more than sentimental good wishes. Many speak of how much I have given to others and how important I have been to art therapy.

I have been holding an image of the hospital machine—a huge maw that will chew me up and spit me out—but now I am going into surgery with confidence. It's bizarre to be feeling well and letting people cut me up, certain that the hysterectomy will be the end of this, no more treatment, no more fears. Maybe I have become my brother, Mr. De-

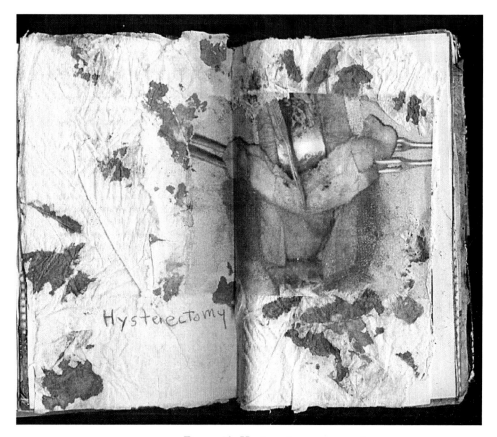

Figure 10. Hysterectomy.

nial, like Sonny. How does he do it, hang in there and stay cheerful? Has my cancer been caught in time? Or is it the sword of Damocles?

A couple of young women surgeons who will assist come in. They are very nice. I go into surgery believing that all will be well.

DAY AFTER SURGERY, JUNE 6

I am connected to beeping instruments–IV [intravenous], oxygen, heart monitor–I don't know what else. I am foggy, but I walk for the first time, just a few steps, gripping the pole that holds all the machinery connected to me. My incision hurts, and trying to walk tires me. I keep pushing the morphine pump, which is supposed to shoot me up every eight minutes, but it doesn't.

The good part is the news. It is great! Rodriguez tells me the surgery showed no evidence of cancer spread. The ovaries were clear, and he even stopped removing lymph nodes before he expected to because all thirty-seven he took out were perfectly clear.

JUNE 7

Neena left early last night. She has the freedom to choose to go home and get a good night's sleep. I feel abandoned. I am totally helpless. I can't get out of bed. I need assistance with everything. Beryl, the heavy nursing assistant, tells me that if I am depressed it will take longer to get well. I know she is right.

My usually low blood pressure was 162 this morning, now it's 140 something. My art supplies are on the other side of the room where I can't get to them. I recline in a chair though. A little act of heroism. I can actually do something for myself.

JUNE 8

I'm confused. I don't know what has happened on what days. The time in the hospital is all a jumble, and it seems so much longer than just a few days. I think about my parents a lot. My poor little Mommy, what could dementia have been like for her?

Visualize healing.

I'm up every half hour to pee. Annoying. I have to get help each time. Sometimes no one comes. I have an "accident" and yell at the nurse for making me wait half an hour before coming. She says no one else was on duty.

The resident tells me I can go home tomorrow, but I'm not ready. I still can't eat or poop. I'm walking better though.

On the phone, Sonny and a former student, Rachel, say that chemo is "nasty stuff." I pray I won't need it.

"My cousin isn't the same person since she's had chemo," Rachel says. Does she want to make me more fearful than I am already? This has all been so sudden. I don't want to live in Cancer Alley. Neena talks about trips we'll take to make me think I'll have a life. Over the phone, my daughter Lisa takes me on a sweet guided imagery trip.

Gradually, I am being disconnected from all the beeping boxes, bags, and tubes that have been hanging off of me, and the nursing staff is becoming more casual in my treatment, even letting me pee by myself.

A large nursing assistant has been bossing me around. When I call Beryl, another nursing assistant, "my main man," she eases off and starts being very nice to me. Jealousy on the surgical unit?

A tall man is racing around the ward pulling his IV pole behind him. I ask him what he's in for. Diverticulitis surgery. He's running in order to poop so he can be discharged.

CANCER ALLEY, JUNE 9

Rodriguez says during surgery they rinse the abdominal cavity with a saline solution to see what they find in the "washings." Mine came out positive: cancer cells. Ten percent of women with uterine cancer have this, he says. Rodriguez is a great one for statistics. Do they mean anything to me? I don't know. Also cancer cells in the omentum, a layer of fat over the intestine. He shakes his head. He doesn't know how they got there. He seems to be talking to himself, "Maybe through the fallopian tubes," he adds. He wasn't going to tell me just yet, he says, but since I asked he had to. What did I ask?

"How can you stand being an oncologist, working with people in terror?" I blurt out.

"It's a privilege to treat them when they are so vulnerable. I want to be of service. I pray a lot." He moves toward the door. "You'll have many more years," his exit line. I doubt that he believes it.

It has spread! I'll be living in Cancer Alley.

I have no time to assimilate the devastating news. Judith and Claire come in the minute Rodriguez leaves. Claire is upset when I tell them. Neena returns from her lunch with Donna, and J & C think we might need some time alone, but Neena wants to know right away what's going on so I tell her. She does not seem phased at all. All the rest of the day she is distant, concerned with the discharge planning and getting some help for herself at home. I've told her to make all the decisions, but she keeps bothering me with them. She maintains that she has more trouble walking than I do and more gas pains. Maybe she is

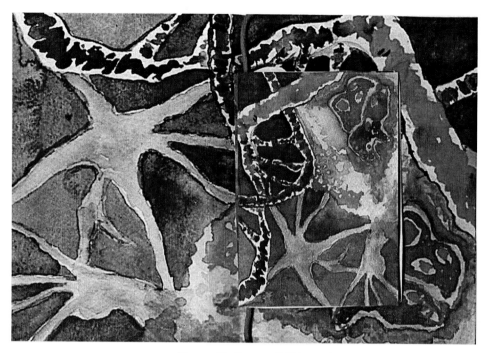

Figure 11. Cancer DNA.

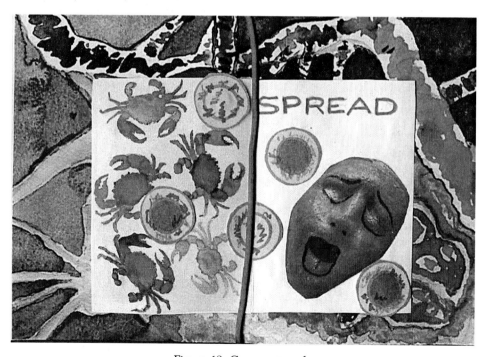

Figure 12. Cancer spread.

trying to push away the impact of the spread of my cancer.

I dread going home and it may be today. The resident tells me the pain medication constipates, so I have to choose.

Helen visits. Her partner Marjorie lived seven years after her ovarian cancer diagnosis. Gail W. calls. Her father never recovered from having his bladder removed because of cancer at this same hospital, but her husband Jim survived lymphoma and bone cancer. It's been five years now. She tells me to get a PET [position emission tomography] scan at Highland Park Hospital. Evanston Hospital doesn't have one.

I'm frightened and depressed. I had been exhilarated that the CAT scan showed no tumors and that nothing was found in the surgery. Maybe I would be safe after all, but it's these invisible insidious crabby buggers that can kill me. I'll have to have chemo and radiation, nausea and debilitation. Cancer Alley is a dark and scary place.

KIDS

Eric's flip buoyancy about how his positive thinking has made me cancer free has become too much, so I tell him about the abdominal washings. I can't bring myself to tell Lisa and Keith. Lisa sends me a large box of all sorts of scented things. She had asked what I wanted and I said lavender lotion, but she sends much more. It is as though she can do something to make it all better. Eric must have told her about the cancer spread because she calls Neena and I tell Neena to tell her. Keith keeps asking when I'll get the pathology report, but I don't say anything about it. I don't want to discuss it with him.

Every time Rachel calls, she asks when my kids are coming in. "If it were my mother, I would be there in a heartbeat." She is around their age and seems to be saying, poor me not to have a daughter like her. I don't want my kids to come. I don't want to be concerned about them. Lisa offered to come as soon as I was diagnosed. I told her not to.

GOING HOME, JUNE 10

They kick me out of the hospital. Insurance isn't going to pay any more than it has to. Judith and Claire help us, carrying all the junk, watering the plants, going to the grocery store—very kind of them.

Margherita comes over with her son—a cute twenty-year-old—to carry up the cripple equipment from my hip replacements that are stored in the basement. A hospital bed is delivered and set up in the dining room.

JUNE 11

I have a horrible backache, probably from the hospital bed, which is much more primitive than the one in the hospital. Neena slept on the living room couch last night because I wanted her nearby. She continues to be sweet to me. I don't know what I'd do if I had to go through this alone.

A home health care nurse from Australia comes. I like her. She tells me her life story, which includes giving up a child for adoption. Gail R. drives two hours to get here, bringing loads of food for many

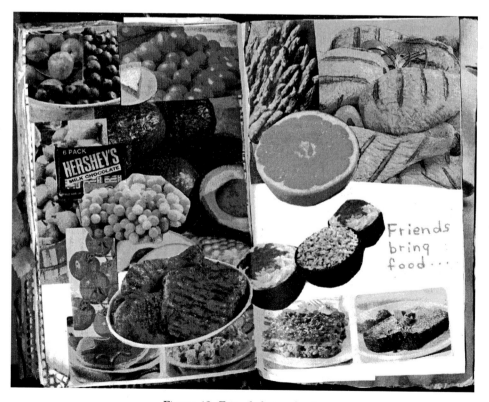

Figure 13. Friends bring food.

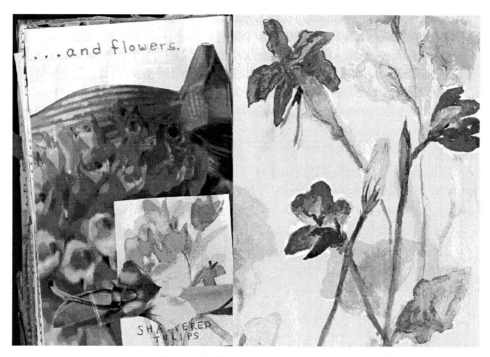

Figure 14. Friends bring flowers.

meals. After Gail leaves, Andra comes with a chicken. She and Neena discuss publishing. I'm glad because I am finding it hard to make conversation. Carolyn comes with more goodies. Joanna and Ellen bring flowers.

Rachel calls and when I tell her I'll probably have to have chemo, once again she tells me how horrible it is. "Your bones will hurt." Thanks a lot, Rachel.

JUNE 12

Last night I awoke unable to breathe because expanding my chest to take a breath hurt so much. Coughing hurts my incision too. Walking hurts my back. I think the hospital bed is breaking my spine. Because my back is killing me, I try to take a nap in my own bed, but the incision hurts too much for me to lie on my side. I'm going to sleep in my own bed anyway. Everyday I have to inject my thigh with an anticoagulant. I hate it.

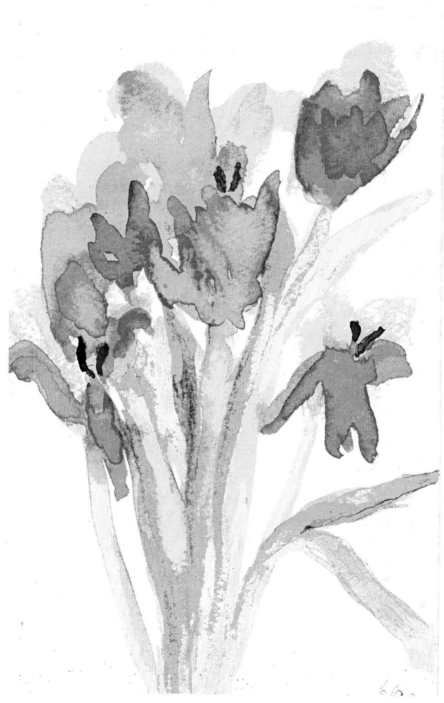

Figure 15. "Shattered Tulips."

I take up my paints for the first time and make several pictures of the tulips that Vicky brought me. They didn't interest me for a painting until they started falling apart. "Shattered Tulips," I call them. Identification? Painting is so good for me. I write thank you notes this evening. That so many people care has made a huge difference.

EIGHTY PERCENT, JUNE 15

I've been thinking about my Pap tests. Maybe I am lucky that I didn't get the results of the one I had a year ago; otherwise I would not have asked Stewart to do this last one, and the cancer would not have been found until it started generating symptoms. Maybe just the opposite: perhaps the Pap test a year ago would have caught the cancer before it spread. My life hangs by a hair. . . .

I see Rodriguez and he floods me with information. Somewhere among all the details of treatment and its effects, he says that if I have no treatment I'll be dead in a year. I think I hear him right. With or without treatment, there is an 80 percent chance of recurrence. I ask him what's the point? "Did I say that?" he responds as though 80 percent is nothing. Recurrence would most likely come in the first few years. He continues: I'll need six treatments of chemo, one every three weeks, Taxol® and Carboplatin, and three sessions of radiation, once a week. He soft-pedals the side effects of chemo, but after he leaves, Ann, the nurse, emphasizes them. She hands me printouts of the details. I'm numb. At home I read them. They describe nausea, vomiting, bruising, bleeding, infection, fatigue, hair loss, sore mouth and bleeding gums, numbness in fingers and toes, rash, itching, and dizziness.

Am I crazy? I am letting people cut me up, poison me, and irradiate me. No, I'm not just letting them, I have asked them to butcher me. I am paying them to torture me. As far as I could tell, nothing was wrong with me. I was feeling no different from how I usually feel. A lab test indicates cancer cells. My doctor tells me that if I don't get treatment I will be dead in a year. Why should I believe any of this? I've been brainwashed. I am crazy.

Another home nurse comes, not the nice woman from Australia. She tries to cheer me up—really lame. She tells me I have been strong all my life (she just met me) so I should be strong now, and of course that I believe in God. When I say no, that stops her.

May 27 was my abrupt banishment to Cancer Land. Today I'm whisked to its center city–"high grade" aggressive cancer that will most likely spread in the next few years. I try to convince myself to enjoy the time I have now. I don't have cancer pain. That may not be the case in the future.

I dig out hats for when I become hairless.

DEATH

Death marched into my consciousness the moment of diagnosis. A stranger I did not know or expect curled up beside me. Because I'd done such a good job of choosing my parents, that stranger had always been remote. My father died at ninety-five, not from the heart failure he had then but from aspirating a piece of food in the nursing home. My mother died at ninety-three. In many ways she was in good health, but she had dementia and refused to eat in the nursing home. She died of starvation. Neither had health problems throughout their long lives until close to the end. How could I have a better pedigree?

I think about what may be my very short road to death and recall a visit with my cousin Harriett in the DC area several years ago. She was ninety-one and had finally stopped being a blonde, surrendering to her natural gray hair, still stylishly coifed. We had lunch in the elegant dining room of her retirement community at Ft. Belvior, VA, for army brass. When I visited her husband, my cousin Bernie, at the nursing home there, she would introduce me as "the General's cousin." I had visited them at their various stations, including Germany, where Bernie was the commandant, so everyone sucked up to me as they did to him. It was a kick. Bernie and Harriett were "the beautiful people," he a handsome proud peacock of a man and she a petite beauty. I had a very special relationship with each of them, doing the dove-hawk thing with Bernie during Vietnam and hearing confidences from Harriett. It was heart-breaking to see Bernie's long, slow decline to complete dependence on Harriett at the end of his life.

At lunch, Harriett was her usual perky self, but she conjectured that at ninety-one she probably wouldn't live more than a couple of years. "My mother died at ninety-three," she said, "and I don't expect to live longer than that."

I wondered what it would be like to be so close to the end of life, to see your life narrow into a funnel of days. How could she decide how to spend her time with so little left? She was living as she always had, playing bridge, getting her hair done, playing the piano for religious services at her residence, where the priest always thanked "the nice little New England Jewish girl" for the music.

I never saw her again, although I talked to her on the phone several times during the week that she died. She was ninety-three.

I talked to my old friend Adele in Rochester, NY, a few days before she died too. I hadn't seen her in years or been in touch except through Christmas cards. One year I didn't receive a card and had a dream about her, so I called. I knew she had been battling breast cancer for thirteen years. In her usual straight-forward way, she told me she was dying, that she had been given two months. Almost speechless, I asked her how she felt about her life. "I've had a very good life," she said. She asked me to send her a picture so she could see how I looked now, and then she had to end the call because a hospice worker had just arrived. I sent the picture, but I doubt she ever saw it. She died two days later. A few years afterwards, her husband Lyman died of cancer as well. During the many years we all lived in the DC area, Lyman and Adele had been very close friends. Lyman Wynne, a psychiatrist renowned for his research in family studies, was a colleague as well. He had secured me my thirteen-year position at the National Institutes of Health (NIH) and had written the forward to my first book (Wadeson, 1980).

There have been too many others. Especially Tory. She had just turned fifty-three when she died of ovarian cancer after fighting it as aggressively as she could for five years. We had lived together for six years, and though twenty years my junior, she had been very much in love with me. She had moved to Michigan in recent years, so I saw her seldom. When we talked, she asked my advice about doing research to get tenure at Purdue where she was teaching or whether she should just live it up in the time she had left? In one call she said, "Claire, this is a horrible disease." Her answering machine didn't work, so sometimes I called her partner Sharon, who lived in Chicago, nearer to me.

A couple months after Tory had told me that the two of them were planning a trip to Baja to see the whales, I left a message for Sharon, saying I was trying to reach Tory. She called back to tell me that Tory had died in the hospital with blood clots in her lungs three days before.

"I want to go," she had told Sharon.

The nurses thought she wanted to go to sleep, but Sharon knew what she meant and told her that she had taken care of everything she had wanted to, "everything is perfect, so you can go." When Sharon returned from getting some supper half an hour later, Tory was dead. She was such a beautiful, spirited person. I never saw her wasted.

I didn't see Harriett, Adele, or Tory waste away, but I was in attendance as my husband's mother, Mema, disintegrated from being a beautiful woman with every hair in place, long manicured fingernails, and designer clothes set off with expensive jewelry, to a skeleton who could no longer speak. During the week of the death vigil around her hospital bed, the family hovered over her or spoke together about funeral arrangements in the small waiting room a few doors down the hall. In her last days at home, Mema hadn't let any of her many friends visit because she didn't want them to see her no longer beautiful, so it was just the family with her at the end.

Lying in the hospital bed, she made smacking sounds with her lips that Aunt Tillie said was her way of trying to kiss us. But I didn't think so. She was beyond that. I doubted that she was aware of anything other than physical sensations. Her mouth was dry, I thought, so I fed her tiny ice chips to wet her lips and mouth. She seemed to like that. It was cancer, of course.

Cancer claimed the lives of almost all of the men with whom I was involved after my divorce; Paul, Charlie, Darrel. They all died miles away, years after our relationships had ended. I read about Paul and Charlie's deaths in the *New York Times* obituary section. Paul was a well-known photojournalist, and Charlie Janeway was a renowned immunologist, president of the Federation of American Societies for Experimental Biology and author of a classic tome on immunology. His research was on T cells in cancer. At a class I was teaching in California, I asked a student who was from Ukiah, where Darrel had moved, if she knew him. She told me of his death. Now I relive special moments I had with each of them and find it hard to imagine them long dead.

I think about my precursors: my father at ninety-five, lying in the nursing home bed for months, not reading or watching TV. I asked him what he was thinking about and he said, "my condition." In my last conversation with him, though, he did manage a bad joke about a talking dog in a bar.

My mother was eating fine when I moved her to the nursing home; in fact, she was still packing it in when they were clearing the lunchroom for bingo. She was a small woman, only five feet tall, and in those last days, she was like my little girl. I walked her outside to see the flowers, I cut her meat for her, I painted her pictures. After spending several days in Washington getting her settled in the nursing home, I left for a month to give workshops in Korea and Japan. I didn't know she had stopped eating soon after I had left.

My mother's death ravaged me. If only I could have talked with her. I would have helped her die, if that was what she wanted. She couldn't remember anything, she probably didn't even know I was her daughter. How could she remain steadfastly determined to die? Lisa, who lives in the DC area, visited her frequently in the nursing home, but in the end she died alone on the one weekend Lisa didn't come. I felt that I had failed her. I seemed to be the only one who could reach her through her dementia. I should have helped her die. I should have been with her.

I had always expected to live at least into my nineties, like my parents. My own death was not a close companion. No one in the family had had cancer, not parents, or uncles and aunts, many who were long-lived. Except my brother, who has been fighting renal cancer for fourteen years. I attribute that to the recent revelation of the toxic dump beneath the park where he played tennis several times a week for years. (His daughter is preparing a class-action suit on behalf of the large number of people in their neighborhood who've gotten cancer.) Recently Sonny collapsed while doing yard work in 100-degree heat and had to be rushed to the emergency room. His wife Joan fights with him about driving the car. He won't give in. He refuses to believe his body is failing him, and he is still upbeat, claiming to be the most fortunate person alive. Cheerily he says of whatever horrible treatment he is undergoing, "It beats the alternative." I wonder. I would have succumbed to depression long ago.

My own death comes crashing in on me. Here I am, like my cousin Harriett, seeing the end in sight. Even at seventy-eight, my horizons had seemed distant. Suddenly, they have clamped shut. The oncolo-

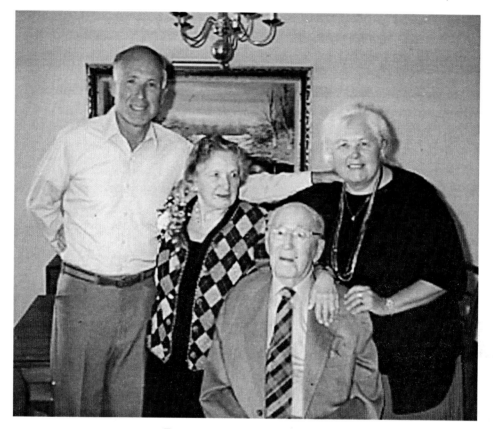

Figure 16. Last family portrait.

gist has told me I have an 80 percent chance of recurrence, most likely in the first years. So I'll have a few years, if I am lucky. Harriett was living her life as she always did, and I suppose I will too (except for the damn treatments). I have done most of what I have wanted to do. I am glad I didn't wait until retirement to travel. I've made a name for myself, trained hundreds of therapists, published lots of books and papers, received awards and honors, helped some people through therapy, and enjoyed my own creativity. My two granddaughters are a delight, and my three children are doing well. I am close to them. I worry about my loss to them, but that will have to come to them sometime. I would like to get my novels published, I would like them to make a splash–that would be a kick–but really only icing on the cake. I have always wanted love, and now it has taken cancer to make me feel I have it, not only from Neena and my children, but from many friends I never knew cared about me as much.

What I am saying is that I think I can go without regret. I don't believe in an afterlife. This is it, and this is enough. For years, I have lived in a state of awe. I marvel at the incredible beauty and intricacy of this world. I place a geranium on my breakfast table so I can watch its buds grow, unfold, and unfurl their petals. I look at the night sky and try to visualize galaxies vaster than my imagination, spiraling ever outwards. I click this computer and wonder how people can make a tiny metal chip hold an entire book.

I reread *Aubade* by Philip Larkin (2003) about his sleepless nights dreading death:

> . . . That this is what we fear—no sight, no sound,
> No touch or taste or smell, nothing to think with,
> Nothing to love or link with. . . .

He died in 1985 at sixty-three.

My dread is not in death, but in dying. I've seen others suffer. When I visited my grandfather as a teenager, he said my sweet gentle grandmother was screaming in her bed from the shingles that were torturing her. They were going to give her a lobotomy, but she died before they could. I've had shingles, but I was lucky to get treated right away. The last time I saw Neena's brother, a very nice, gentle person with prostate cancer, he had become bitter over his misdiagnosis and the suffering he was enduring. He said, "Why can't I just get this over with?"

Eighty percent chance of recurrence. I'll either beat this thing or fall into that large 80 percent pit. I know of others who are going from treatment to treatment, more surgeries, constant chemotherapy. I don't want to be there. I think of suicide as my safety net. Will I have the courage to do it while I am still capable? I need to keep the car filled with gas, I keep thinking, fearful that when the time comes, I may be too debilitated to do so. As spring blossoms around me, I recall a clear October day when the blazing sugar maples of Door County ignited my eyes, and I don't see how I will ever be able to leave such beauty. Then I sink back again into the quagmire of dread.

Death creeps around the corner on soft cat feet with a sad smile. "I'll hold you," she whispers. "I'll end all your suffering."

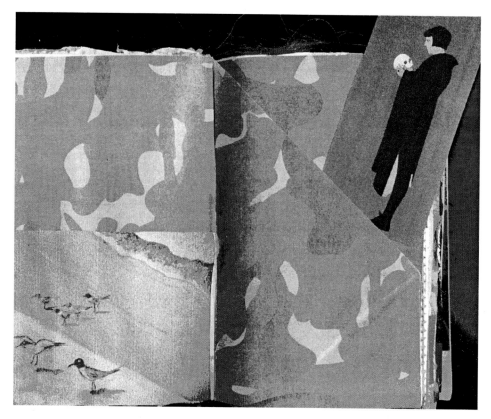

Figure 17. Death.

JUNE 17, 18

I have horrible conversations, first with Roberta, an old friend from our young married years. She leaves me dangling on the phone while she gets her hearing aids. After a reasonable amount of time, I hang up. She calls back and complains about her arthritis and over and over about the two wonderful e-mails she sent me that I should look for, but not a word asking how I am. Janet calls—not a word of compassion from her either, just that she rushed out to get a Pap test. She doesn't seem to know what else to say, and Janet is a social worker with lots of clinical experience. Then there's Rachel, who calls every day to tell me how chemo will hurt my bones.

Most people are kind and considerate though. Claire S. and Margherita offer to drive me to chemo. What I've learned: the most important attribute is kindness. I used to go for intellect and creativity, perceptiveness, sensitivity. It's so much more simple. Just kindness.

Is dread the worst thing? Dread of the D&C report when Swenson had called me in early, dread that the CAT scan would show tumors elsewhere, dread of the surgery pathology report? Dread is a horror, terror. Now I have dread of chemo, dread of a recurrence. Probably dread is not the worst thing. Pain and suffering are worse.

I am recovering from surgery. I can move better and there is less pain, although my back still aches and impairs my walking.

Judith and Claire call. Claire tells me that their friend Claudia has been diagnosed with ovarian cancer that has spread, but Claire feels good about me. I've been getting e-mail responses to my latest announcement—everyone is happy about my good news. Am I crazy? I wrote that I feel hopeful because there has been no spread to lymph nodes or organs. I didn't send out an e-mail after I got news of the spread of cells to my abdomen and omentum.

The kit from the American Cancer Society tells me stage III uterine cancer has a 30 percent five-year survival rate and that my brand, serous papillary carcinoma, is the fast-spreading kind of uterine cancer with a poorer prognosis. It can spread to the bladder and rectum. More dread.

I feel better however when Gail R. comes over, and we have fun searching through basement boxes for wigs and hair. I don't know if they are usable. People are still bringing food. The kitchen is crammed with it, and there is a continuous display of flowers all over the house. Judith and Claire bring a lovely salmon dinner, along with a bit too much cross-examination. I know it comes from their interest and concern, but sometimes I just don't want to talk about cancer.

LISA'S BIRTHDAY, JUNE 21

My daughter Lisa decides at the last minute to spend her birthday with me, so she and her husband Mark fly in from Virginia, which is a big challenge because Lisa is afraid of flying. It's really nice of them in the midst of their busy lives with many arrangements to make in order to be gone. Lisa is very affectionate. Mark is sweet and mops up our flooded basement for us.

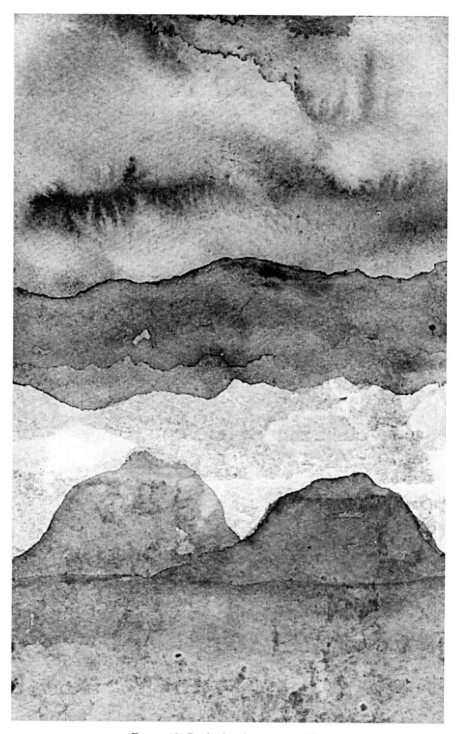

Figure 18. Dark clouds over my life.

We walk around the Northwestern lagoon and have an elegant birthday dinner at Jilly's, a small restaurant near our house with very good food. But I still have post-surgical digestion complications. After dinner I have cramps from constipation. I'm miserable. Rocks that won't come out. I have to dig them out with a plastic glove. Disgusting! Then when I am showing Lisa and Mark slides of our recent trip to Patagonia, I have to dash to the bathroom where I explode with diarrhea that pushes out the constipation. I go upstairs to change my clothes and wash them while feeling horrible. No one comes to see what's wrong with me. Later I try to explain what was happening to me to Neena, but she can't understand, for reasons that I can't understand.

JUNE 22, 23

Lisa sleeps late, so it's okay that I have an early appointment to go to the hospital to have the surgery staples removed. Since Rodriguez is on vacation, I see his female associate whom I had wanted to treat me in the first place. She asks me what the incision was for. When I tell her I had a hysterectomy, she asks what that was for. "Uterine cancer," I reply. You'd think she could take a minute to look at the chart of a patient she is seeing for the first time! I'm glad she's not my doctor. She leaves and Ann removes the staples. What was the point of having an appointment with the doctor in the first place?

We go to the Botanic Gardens, and Mark pushes me around in a wheelchair so I am able to see much more than I would otherwise. He and Lisa love it.

We order Indian food delivered for dinner, and Neena, who has been on edge through much of their visit, yells at Mark for asking about taking a large piece of *naan.*

"That is no way to talk to someone," he bristles. He is usually a mild-mannered, considerate guy, but he pushes away from the table in anger and goes upstairs. Lisa follows him.

I'm furious at Neena, "You're making me sick," I spit out at her.

"I'm bearing the brunt of everything."

"No. I am."

I go upstairs and apologize to Mark for her. He's nice about it and comes back downstairs. Neena apologizes. Later she and Mark have a long talk, and she apologizes again. I think she is resentful that Lisa has not offered to help.

I know my children love me. It will be hard on them if a die soon.

After Lisa and Mark leave for the airport, Ellen comes over and tells me about the Sweden trip that I was supposed to lead, the trip I'd forsaken to have surgery. Everyone had a great time. They spoke of me often, she says, and they all think I'm wonderful. I'm like a goddess to them, she adds. Jill, my Australian colleague for whom I have taught many times, told her I saved her life. I had consulted in her establishing art therapy training there. The Sweden trip sounds marvelous. I'm glad, but sorry I missed it.

JEWISH HAIR

My hair is my signature. Friends use it to spot me in a crowd. It's shiny white and long and thick, held in place by one of my many barrettes at the nape of my neck and cascading down my back like a torrential waterfall. Chemo will make it all fall out.

Goldie from my novel writing group is a member of an orthodox Jewish community in which married women wear wigs, like my great grandmother did. Goldie's wig is golden and beautiful. If I hadn't been told, I never would have suspected that it was not her natural hair. I don't know Goldie very well, but I ask her if she can recommend a wig maker. Since I have a lot of hair, I have decided to have a wig made from my own hair, so in a way I won't lose it after all. Goldie tells me her wig maker is the best in the Mid West and offers to drive me to her house, where she runs her business out of her basement. Goldie is very gracious. She is getting a new wig and suggests that I watch so I can have an idea of how it all works. We drive to the West Rogers Park area of Chicago, where there is an enclave of Hasidic Chabad-Lubavitch Jews. The small ranch and split-level houses are 1950s models. The women, including Goldie, wear skirts to their ankles and long sleeves. Men and boys wear yarmulkes, and men don't shave, so most have gray full beards, totally unshaped.

Chaya Sara is a lovely woman with a scarf around her head who makes me feel right at home amidst all the wigs lying on the table and perched on stands with faces crowding shelves lining the wall. All are human hair. She and Goldie rave about my hair, and when I unclip the barrette and it falls around my shoulders, they gasp. We have girl time, chatting while Chaya Sara shapes Goldie's wig.

It's time for me to bite the bullet. They ask if I want to think it over, but I tell Chaya Sara to chop away. She lines up my shorn locks on a table, and her two-year-old daughter comes in. I worry that she might grab some of the hair and mess it up, but she doesn't. The hair will be sent off to be made into a wig, a *sheitel,* as they call it. The conceit of having a wig made from my own hair will cost me $2500 because each hair has to be woven in singly. I need this indulgence right now.

I thought I would be like Samson, disempowered with my hair cut off, but actually I like it. It's about an inch long all over. Neena loves it. She thinks I look butch.

Sitting in our back room watching TV, Neena melts into a smile, "You look so beautiful with your hair short. I love you, Claire."

When we have dinner with our monthly potluck group in the lovely backyard at the home of one of them, everyone raves about my hair the whole evening, not just when they first see me. I guess I look like most of them with short white hair. Rachel comes over the next day and says I look like a *bubbe* (grandma). I can do without that.

I get bizarre e-mails from my brother Sonny and his wife Joan in response to the picture I sent them of me with shorn hair. He says he's glad I no longer look like a witch and now resemble our mother more, and she says short hair should be cool for the summer. Right! Very cool–I'll lose it all! Then she wishes me a nice summer. Right again. I'm sure chemo summers are just great.

Chaya Sara calls and says the wig will be too expensive as originally planned, so they are going to send it to Brazil to be made. She needs to take measurements of my head right away so they can start immediately. They will complete it in about a month instead of the usual two months. Neena drives me to Chaya Sara's, where measuring takes five minutes. Then we spend the next two hours talking, about her having gone to Australia because the *Rebbe* had told her to, her arranged marriage, finding a suitable husband for her special needs daughter, her beliefs, her wish to move to Israel where she is expecting the Messiah to come very soon. Although she is already a grandmother with six children, Chaya Sara is only forty-two. I learn about the Lubavitches and their mission to reach out to other Jews. The dis-

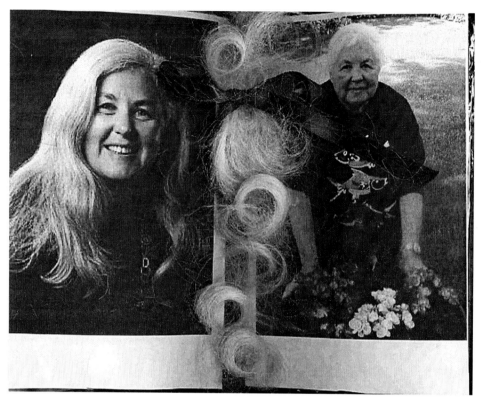

Figure 19. Before and after haircut.

cussion ends with an invitation to Shabbat dinner the following week.

Going to Chaya Sara's house for dinner is like entering a home in Eastern Europe 100 years ago. The living room is dark with large furniture and a wall of shelves holding *menorahs,* Jewish figurines, and books. The dining room table is set elaborately with white linen and a zillion candles, and the chairs are dressed in garnet slipcovers. Friends and family are coming and going. The men are dressed in black suits, some with sashes, and old-fashioned broad-brimmed black hats. The women light the candles on the table, a large silver candelabra and many smaller candles. Chaya Sara says the blessing, welcoming the Sabbath queen, and we all pray for what we want. (Guess what I pray for!) Two boys are running around and bang into the glass door of the living room bookcase and shatter it. No one seems too upset. The men leave for *shule,* and the women visit in the living room. They are very interested in art therapy, but have rigid ideas about interpretation, including Chaya Sara's mother, who is a therapist.

When the men return, we go to the table, where they say prayers and drink wine. There is an abundance of cold dishes, which I think is the meal, so I fill up. They clear away the dishes and bring out chicken, meat, potatoes, and two kinds of *kugel*. For dessert, there is a carrot birthday cake for one of the friends.

Of course, Neena has to be her scientist self and her provocateur self by challenging Chaya Sara's husband, stating that modern-day genetics can now determine that a child with a Jewish father and a non-Jewish mother carries Jewish genes. He responds that God has decreed that a child's religion is determined by its mother. It's written in the *Torah*. Neena brings up evolution, which is like a firecracker, and the response is to pooh-pooh Darwin because "scientists are always changing their minds." The earth is a certain age (somewhere around 7,000 years, according to The Law), and that's that.

If my leg were longer, I would kick Neena under the table. You don't argue faith, especially with the host when you are a guest at his table. I say something about the importance of respecting other people's beliefs and shift to observing that whatever people in Thailand and Bali believe, they live out their beliefs so that you never ever hear a voice raised in anger there, which certainly isn't true in this country or Israel. We need to respect that and maybe even learn from it, I say. I don't think anyone is too upset. They all seem to enjoy asserting themselves, and arguing points of belief appears to be their custom. One of the guests, Faygie, wants us to come to them too, but maybe changes her mind after hearing Neena.

On the way home, Neena says that they were trying to convert her. I don't feel that at all. I love entering this foreign community, so close and yet so distant from me, in the same way I love exploring other cultures in my travels. I wonder if my ancestors were like them.

JUNE 24–26

We're sweating in a heat wave. Level of gratification: I have a normal poop this morning.

Judith and Claire come over. Claire brings a cancer book by Keith Block (2009). She's all excited about his nutritional program. I read it and crash into depression. I can't do this.

After Toyan, the bath lady, comes and Mark, the physical therapist, discharges me, Neena and I have trouble finding the American Cancer Society office, where we are going to pick up the free wig they give to cancer patients. I try on wigs. They are scratchy and tight, made from synthetic hair. I look hideous in all of them. Finally I choose one that I think is the least ugly, which they give me along with some knitted hats, also to cover my soon-to-be-bald head. The woman helping me is very nice, and it is a good service.

JUNE 27

Lisa is writing me a poem each day. They are very sweet. Hearing about Lisa's daily poems, Keith begins sending me a photo each day, mostly of his kitchen rehab work.

Tony, a former student and the assistant my publisher gave me a stipend to pay to help me with the art therapy book I am revising, comes over and we work on the book. It's a drag that drags me down. Him too, I think. He's a fun, spirited guy, but even he can get flagged from the tedium of numbering and coordinating more than 100 pictures with the text.

I continue to struggle to formulate a diet, one that will be healthful and that I will be able to tolerate once I begin chemo. Block's book (2009) has lots of suggestions, but I don't like most of the foods he recommends. I have a long talk with friend and colleague Nancy S. about it. She has been a vegetarian for thirty years.

Big night on the town (my last pre-chemo) with Judith and Claire. We have dinner at Petterinos next to the Goodman Theatre. Neena is unusually quiet and very affectionate toward me, but she has problems with Claire's attachment to alternative medicine and makes a snide comment about "real medicine." Claire flares. I am sitting between the two of them and try to make peace. I don't need people fighting around me with me in the middle. Earlier Neena told me that my interest in Claire's advice and in organic foods is a "repudiation" of all she believes in. She considers it flakey. Her identity as a scientist (a reproductive biologist) is iron clad.

The play at the Goodman is good, but at the end the husband is a helpless double amputee whose wife does everything for him. I don't need to see that.

On the way home, Judith and Claire talk about how Claudia is dealing with ovarian cancer. She is having a presurgery party and getting biofeedback. She seems so much more on top of getting herself taken care of than I am. General Claudia has also marshaled her troops: Mattie is to pick up the family at the airport. Silvia, Ben, and Maria have been recruited for chemo chauffeuring. Ginnie is detailed to researching the new smart phone Claudia's partner Bev wants to buy for her. Claudia's friends have been notified that they are to give her only positive messages.

"Claudia sure is the CEO of her disease," I say. Maybe I should be too, but I feel too depleted for all this organizing. More significantly, I don't have the sort of relationships with my friends in which I would feel comfortable in marshaling them in this way.

JUNE 28

I finally work out the shopping list Neena has been asking me to write, and she and I go to Whole Foods. Neena is pissed at Claire for messing up my mind with Block's book. Shopping takes forever because I don't know where anything is. Neena's knee is bothering her and she has to sit down. At the end when I've gotten fatigued, I sit and Neena checks us out. In the elevator to the roof parking lot, she loses it completely, banging the cart against the wall because they wouldn't take a check (from our household account) so she had to use her credit card. She screams that she pays for everything. I tell her I will pay for it all, and she starts yelling about how ridiculous it is to buy organic food. In the car, it finally comes out—no one gave her any attention or helped her out when she was diagnosed with atrial fibrillation. She's envious of me! Competitive as ever. I scream back that I can't stand this and that I will get other people to help me out. It feels good to yell. I notice that when I bark at Neena, I feel better. I've got to get out my anger. There must be a more positive way.

At home, I call Claire and ask her to pick up stuff at Whole Foods for me because Neena has trouble with it. Neena hears me and becomes furious and is not speaking to me. I can't fight cancer and Neena too. It's too much.

Later when I tell Lisa about it, she says that as a safety net I can always come live with her. Ha! Forget my medical treatment and support system? What I would need would be for her to come here. No chance of that.

JUNE 29

The day before chemo. The day before surgery I had thought that it might be the last day I felt fine ever. Today I don't feel fine—horrible constipation—spending most of the afternoon on the toilet with no results. This might be the last day I am not totally miserable.

Neena keeps asking what I want to eat. I think she is getting impatient with me, but she is reigning in her irritation and suggesting foods she thinks I'll like. I so appreciate her trying, but I don't want ANY-THING. I've lost twenty pounds since my diagnosis. Not a diet I would recommend.

D-DAY, JUNE 30

Portal #2, chemo. D-Day, drip day, dread day. But now to get on with it. The heat wave broke in time for my chemo. Neena parks on the roof lot of Evanston Hospital, and we walk the long twisted corridors with their gurneys of sick patients to Elevator E that lets us off at the Kellogg Cancer Center. Sitting in the crowded waiting room, I look over the other patients. A few are in wheelchairs. Some wear hats to cover their bald heads. A technician calls me in to the lab to draw blood to determine if my red and white blood cell counts are high enough to withstand the destruction of chemotherapy. I tell her that my veins are so small I need a child's needle. She says she will use a butterfly needle. Unlike most of the others, she gets it in on the first stick. We take Elevator F down to Rodriguez's office and wait half an hour for him.

He's bright and chipper, but he doesn't even notice that my hair has been cut. He tells me that I look the same. Does he even see me? But worse, he tells me I have an 80 percent chance of a recurrence with or without chemo, with most recurrences coming in the first several years. So what am I doing this for? He says we've gone over this before, but I just didn't get it. I'm confused and frightened. Not a great way to go into chemo. I remind myself that he said without treatment I would be dead in a year.

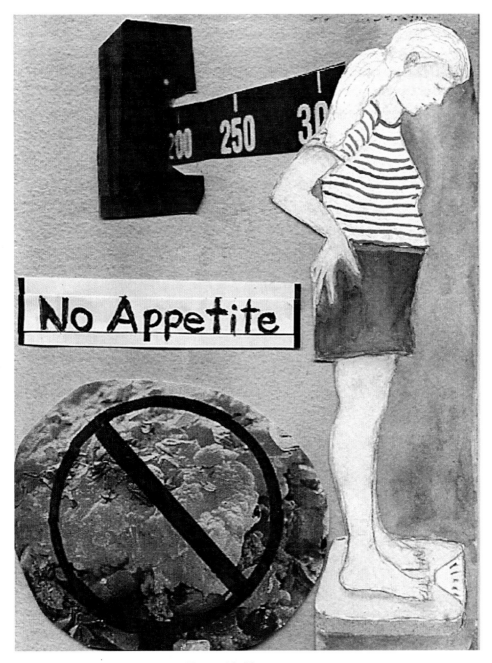

Figure 20. No appetite.

Neena and I go back up the elevator to the hospital's Kellogg Cancer Center, where the nurse Julia leads me to a small private room and seats me in a green La-Z-Boy that replaces the bed. The leg rest shoots out so suddenly it could do damage to anyone standing too close. She attaches the IV to the back of my left hand because I tell her I want to draw with my right one. There are plastic things hanging off the tube and lots of surgical tape. I arrange all the supplies I've brought to entertain myself during the four-hour drip and begin by drawing a picture of my hand with the tube looping into me and fastened with lots of tape and the chemo pole with its machine and bags of poison hanging from it.

I'm too absorbed in drawing to pay much attention to the nurse monitoring the infusion of Taxol to be sure I don't have an allergic reaction. I don't.

Drip, drip, buzz, buzz goes the machine on the IV pole. Bags dripping poison, like the udders of witch cows. Kill those crabby cancer cell suckers. I'll beat this rap.

I'm wearing a blouse that's opened over my T-shirt. I'd taken it off my left arm for all the tubing taped to me. When I have to drag my IV pole with all the paraphernalia hanging from it to the bathroom, moving is a problem. The loosened sleeve drops into the toilet.

Sally, a psychology post-doc young enough to be my granddaughter, comes in and explains other therapies available: acupuncture, massage, meditation, music therapy. I can feel myself sinking into a bog of grog. My words are slow and slurred from the Benadryl® to prevent something, maybe nausea. I sleep in the uncomfortable La-Z-Boy. In addition to pastels, I'd brought a book, my i-Pod, audiobooks, and a CD player. I don't use any of them. I sleep for several hours. Julia unhooks me and says she's writing an order for me to get less Benadryl next time so I won't be knocked out. I've been infused with a saline solution, prednisone, Taxol (for most of the time), and Carboplatin. I go home and sleep some more.

I feel fine. I wash out my blouse that dragged into the toilet, and I empty all the bathroom trash. It's a relief to have the treatment over, but there is the dread of tomorrow and the next day. I'm wearing Sea-Bands and drinking ginger tea, hoping, hoping, hoping not to get nauseous.

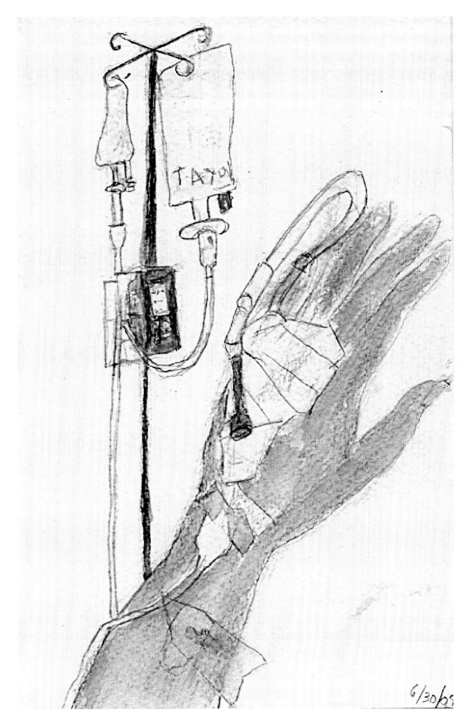

Figure. 21. Drawing during chemo.

DAY AFTER CHEMO, JULY 1

I'm wired from steroids in the drip and couldn't sleep much after 3:30 AM. I feel okay. NO NAUSEA. HOORAY! Cramps and still constipated though.

Rodriguez calls, as well as a Kellogg pharmacist, to see how I am doing on the chemo. I'm really glad that they are thinking about me the day after. I feel cared for and supported. The bath lady Toyan, from Nigeria, and the home nurse Angie, from the Philippines, come today. There are lots of calls to see how I am.

Until now, this memoir has been an illegible scrawl in a notebook. Today I start typing what I have written into the computer.

I have given myself time and space. Time to recover from chemo. Time to do what I want. I have resigned from committees, dropped out of my novel writing group and Aqua Fitness class, and Ruth has agreed to teach my Northwestern University course this month.

In the evening, I'm pooped and feeling sort of sickish.

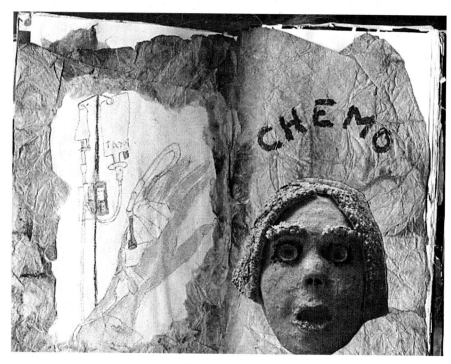

Figure 22. Chemo in the altered book.

JULY 2

Constipation turns into diarrhea. I don't know what meds to take or not. There's a sharp pain in my left hip—oh God, I hope my hip replacement isn't falling apart. At night I have bone aches. I can't sleep. What do I think about? Suicide. I work out how I will communicate it to my kids. Each time I think it over, my plan becomes more refined.

JULY 3

I feel sick all day. Lots of visitors come, and I enjoy talking to them out on the deck, but I get tired. Later I do a painting of chemo capturing cancer cells (crabs) and blood cells with new blood cells coming in, which makes me feel a little better.

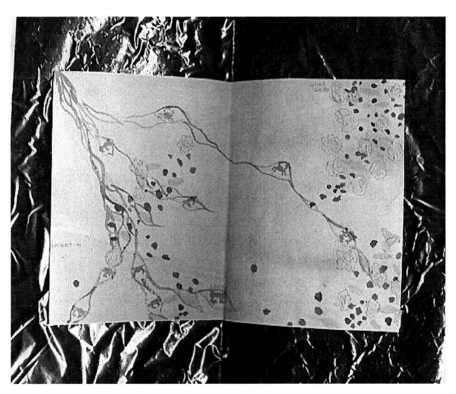

Figure 23. Chemo killing cells.

Judith and Claire report that Claudia had surgery yesterday. She has lots of cancer spread to various organs, though not in them. The surgeon couldn't remove all of it. It doesn't look good.

The chemo blast comes this evening–a sick feeling, stomach cramps, back and leg aches, rapid heart beat, hot but no fever. I'm weak and can hardly walk. I have to lie down. I want to die. I take a sleeping pill.

JULY 4–8

I sleep all morning. I'm exhausted and still have cramps but less leg pain. I cancel the fireworks with Ellie and Cyndi and ask Neena to answer my phone. I don't even talk to Lisa. Poor Neena. She tries to make me feel better and I don't. Will I ever feel better? I don't do anything all day, except sleep some more in the afternoon.

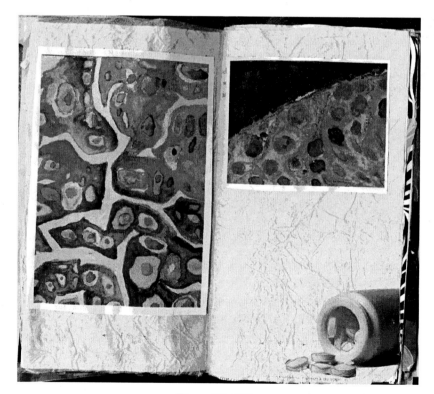

Figure 24. Pills.

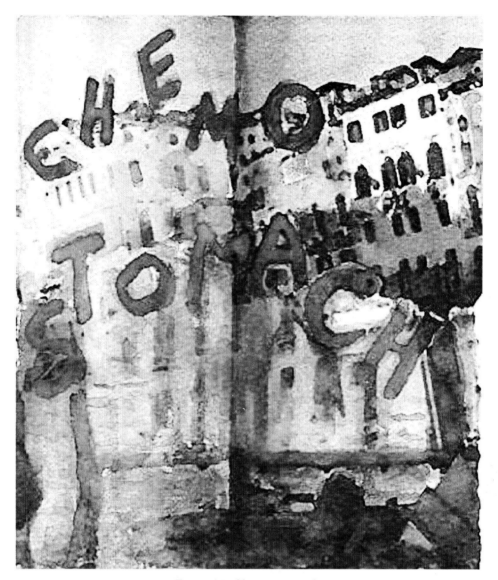

Figure 25. Chemo stomach.

I read *The Adventures of Cancer Bitch* (Wisenberg, 2009). I'm envious that Wisenberg had only stage II cancer, while I have stage III, and that her chemo drip took only thirty minutes, not hours like mine. Right after a treatment she was able to walk three miles. I can hardly walk at all. Her chances of recurrence were 20 percent, not 80 pecent like mine. Her cancer may have all been excised by the surgery. Mine is still here.

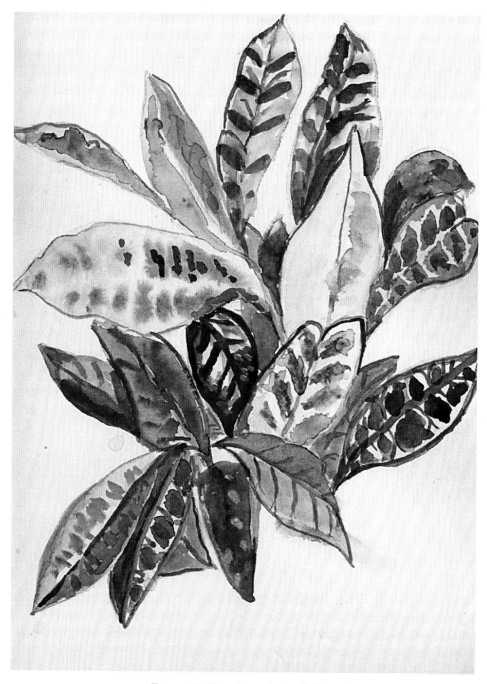

Figure 26. Plant brought by Helen.

I feel a little better, though still sickish, queasy, and weak. I finish *Cancer Bitch*. Maybe I shouldn't be reading about cancer experiences. Poor Neena. She has to do everything. I want to write today, but I can't. I still haven't cried.

Neena wants to watch Agatha Christie's *Miss Marple* on TV. The victims are all killed by the poison taxine, made from yew trees. I'm getting Taxol, made from yew trees. The same poison!

I'm feeling better, but I still can't eat. I'm not building up my blood with protein and extra calories the way I should. More visitors come. I paint two pictures of the plant Helen brought and show her when she arrives.

DIETICIAN, JULY 9

Neena drives me to see an oncology dietician at Evanston Hospital. I'm more confused than ever. I may have been eating all wrong–the bland stuff so I won't be nauseous, like bread and crackers. I've been eating whole wheat and other fiber, which she says may have been causing gas. She tells me to try small amounts of things to see how I react. How can I tell what causes what? I need more protein.

I have blood drawn. All the blood cell counts are down, but not too much, so I don't have to get a white cell booster shot with whatever side effects that may cause. That's a relief.

More visitors. They are a distraction from my depression.

POTLUCK, JULY 11

Early in the day, Rachel visits. She appraises my short curly white hair and squinches up her face, "You look like a *bubbe*."

Well Rachel, I feel like saying, *bubbe* is better than bald, which is what I'll be the next time you see me.

Robinlee comes later and shows me videos of the Sweden trip and brings a gift the Sweden group made in the glass studio, really sweet of them. Apparently, they talked about me a lot. Many have sent nice messages.

Neena and I haven't gone to the monthly potluck group since winter. We go to Joanne's lovely backyard and see folks who haven't come in a long time. I am able to eat most things now. Everyone raves about my short hair all evening, not just when I arrive. It's grown with curls sprouting out from my head. I no longer look butch (if I ever did). My hair feels funny, as though the roots are clutching my scalp. It's been two weeks since my first chemo and my hair hurts.

JULY 12, 13

I've been working on the art therapy book and send off stuff to Isabel, my editor. Neena and I take our longest walk yet, by the Northwestern lagoon with red-winged blackbirds trilling all around us. It's a beautiful clear windy day, and we walk all the way along the lake to the point, where we watch sailboats and wind surfers racing the wind. We sit on a bench and talk with a nice Chinese couple.

My energy is increasing. The kitchen is chaos with all the food people have brought and we have bought, so that I can't find anything in the fridge. I clean it out and reorganize it.

My brother Sonny calls from Connecticut, and we talk about denial. His wife Joan joins in and says he's crazy. I tell him his kids think he is too, but I add that obviously denial works for him so I'm a big fan.

NEENA'S MELTDOWN, JULY 14

We go to the south Whole Foods and Neena gets mad at me because I check us out and she doesn't know where I am, even though I call to her. She has a hearing deficit, so I probably should have gone over to her, but I am fatigued. The kitchen is still chaos, so I reorganize the shelves because there is no room for anything. Neena doesn't like it when I arrange, but I need a little order. I think all the stress is getting to her. She raves away about how she is doing everything for me and she can't stand it anymore. She threatens to walk out. Great! This is all I need. I can't get through this by myself.

MEDITATION AT THE BOTANIC GARDENS, JULY 15

The Cancer Wellness Center is a beautiful facility in Northbrook, about a half-hour drive from my house. At no cost, it provides all kinds of support services for those who have had cancer and their caregivers, such as support groups, yoga, tai chi, educational programs, and much more. I have not felt well enough to drive there, but Claire S. comes with Neena and me to the Botanic Gardens for meditation sponsored by the Cancer Wellness Center. The day is cloudy and breezy–lovely. After seated meditation, we meditate while walking around in the gardens. Walking slowly by myself with no route or destination, just noticing the flowers, the dew drops, the crunching of gravel beneath my feet, is a whole different way of enjoying the garden. Very peaceful. Usually I have a route and try to see as much as I can.

We wipe out all the meditation benefits by going to Costco. On the way home, Neena is in a tizzy because we can't get off the expressway and have to backtrack. When we get home, she starts goading me about my trying to organize the kitchen, and I scream at her. I am not proud of behaving this way. When I get up from my nap, she says she'll die if I don't kiss her. I tell her she has been incredibly cruel.

THE CAREGIVER

I want to tell the truth about my cancer experience. I want to show the whole picture, even the disgusting parts, like my digestive problems. I want to state my fears and anxieties, my ups and downs. This is not a tale of heroics. Living with cancer and undergoing the torment of its treatment is a many-layered experience. Other people play a major role, and the primary caregiver is monumentally important. I don't know what I would do without Neena. Going through such an experience alone would be excruciating for me. I feel so sorry for those who have no choice but to go it alone. To say I appreciate Neena and all she is doing for me is a vast understatement. Just having her here with me, knowing that she cares and that she wants to help me makes all the difference.

The Cancer Wellness Center has a writing group led by Dan, an English teacher who seems very nice. His partner, who died of cancer, wrote pieces to their four-year-old son during his illness, words of wisdom, I suppose. So now Dan is writing for their son too. He is no doubt thinking of his little boy when he gives us an assignment to write about our audience. Well, that just doesn't work for me, because I am writing for myself. Dan says that his partner was very angry and rejected his efforts of help. So I am thinking that is what Dan should be writing about, how difficult it can be for the caregiver. Many people have written about their cancer experience, but I doubt that there is much out there about what life is like for the caregiver.

What a flood of emotions there must be for those who love a cancer sufferer and especially those who are in the position of primary caretaker. No doubt there is grief and sorrow, but so much more as well. Perhaps even joy sometimes in being able to help, especially when the help is appreciated. There must be fatigue from all the effort and resentment at how one-sided it is, and fear, great fear, about what horrors lie ahead, and dread of eventual death and loss. For some, love may deepen. The dimensions of closeness and distance may stretch and shrivel.

Banishment to Cancer Land is not a choice for those who are stricken, but it is for those who take care of them. They must want to bail out at times. In many of the illness memoirs I've read, the caregivers are perfect souls of devotion. I don't believe them.

Neena certainly didn't ask to be my caregiver. Who does? I guess she figures it comes with the territory. She drives me to my appointments and keeps a notebook of questions for the doctor and writes down his answers. Because she is a physiologist who has taught in med schools, she is a valuable source of medical information for me, as well as a resource for medical contacts I need. She tries to prepare food I will like and becomes frustrated because I don't like anything. She asks me what I want for dinner, and I can't tell her because even water tastes bad to me.

Neena is eight-two years old. She has atrial fibrulation for which she must take coumadin every day. She tires easily. She has severe arthritis too, for which she takes a low dose of prednisone. My illness is very trying for her. She doesn't speak about her fears and says she knows I will be fine. Maybe she too sails down de-Nile. But more likely, she suppresses expressions of her anxiety so as not to add to mine.

Caring for me along with what must be anxiety over the seriousness of my illness is taking its toll. Periodically, she loses it. She gets angry that all the care falls to her. I think she wishes my children would carry some of the burden.

Neena is a tightly wound person, and even in the best of times she becomes overwhelmed frequently. She angers easily and blurts out castigations in her frustration. She has been trying very hard to rein in her temper. Sometimes I see her stifle her anger, and at other times she lets it loose. She wants to take care of me and feels like a failure that, try as she may, she can't make me feel better. I tell her that I appreciate all she is doing for me. I tell her I don't see how I could go through this alone. For the most part, she is very sweet to me. I try to show my appreciation, but when she snaps at me, I snap back. Along with my blood cells, nerve cells, and intestinal tract lining, chemo has zapped my patience cells as well.

With medical problems of her own, Neena often becomes overwhelmed by my needs. I am trying to give a full and honest account of my experience, but if she should ever read this, I worry that writing of the difficulties I have with her sometimes will be unkind and unappreciative of all she is doing for me. Will she ever forgive me? Will she desert me?

DAYS IN THE SALT MINE, NIGHTS ON THE TOWN, JULY 16–20

I drive to the grocery store—my first time behind the wheel since surgery. The hospital bed is removed from the dining room. I'm glad to be rid of it. We move the raised toilet seat down to the basement, so the house is no longer a sick bay.

I finally catch up with myself in writing this memoir. Hooray. I make soup, do laundry, take care of plants, all to get ready for my second chemo treatment in two days. For the first time since my diagnosis, I work a little on my novel, *Reading Rebecca.* I like it. Tony and I work our butts off numbering endless pictures for the art therapy book. I am so sick of it. He works on it some more and delivers it the next day and stays for a long visit. I can't tell him I'm too tired to chat.

The day after, which is my last day before chemo—the day I want to send off the art therapy book to the publisher and be done with it—I discover that Tony's computer and mine don't speak the same language, so pictures he worked on are skewed and overly cropped on my computer. I go down to the basement and drag out all the glossy black and whites that accompanied the first edition from the Dark Ages and renumber them. It takes forever. Then I make a disk for the pictures in the nine new chapters and finally get my editor Isabel on the phone. I explain all, and she says the glossies will be fine. That's a relief. I write elaborate instructions and send everything. I think Tony is discouraged, but I try to bolster him.

I finish reading *My Stroke of Insight* (Taylor, 2006) by a neuro-anatomist who had a stroke, thanking her zillions of cells and ending with "Donate your brain to Harvard."

The nights are much better. We have an elegant dinner at Jilly's with David, the husband of Neena's niece, and Max, their son, who are visiting to look over Northwestern University. Then a fantastic night out Saturday. Former student Vicky and her husband Jim take us to a gala performance at Ravinia, a beautiful outdoor pavilion and art deco theater in Chicago's northern suburbs. They bring everything and insist on carrying it all—tables, chairs, food, drinks. We sit outside the pavilion on the extensive lawn where there is hardly a blade of grass to be seen the place is so crowded. The program is exceptional: the Chicago Symphony conducted by James Conlon playing *Fanfare for the Common Man; A Lincoln Portrait,* narrated by Jesse Norman; and *Beethoven's Ninth* with unbelievable soloists and the great Chicago Symphony Chorus. What a treat and so generous of Vicky and Jim. They won't let us do a thing, not even pay for our tickets.

I am wearing the navy slacks, jacket, and hat I bought for Sweden and spend much of the concert picking my rapidly escaping white hairs off my clothes. I see short hairs floating around me before they land, like a cloud of dandelion fuzz.

The night before chemo we go out to dinner at Convito's with Judith and Claire. The evening is beautiful so we sit outside.

CHEMO #2, JULY 21

My blood count is down but high enough to withstand treatment. I'm glad. I don't want it delayed. Rodriguez tells me that I am doing fine. I feel proud of myself for being strong. Reactions to chemo are very individual, he says. Some people go from chemo to their offices. I think they must be getting different chemicals from mine.

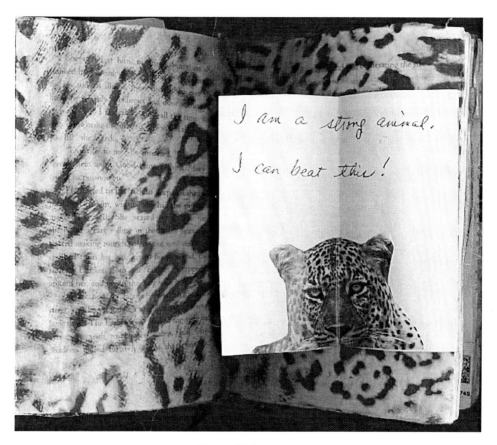

Figure 27. Strength.

This time I talk with Sally, the psychologist, before the drip so I can stay awake. She is affirming but addresses my advanced stage fears by talking about palliative care to prevent "pain and torture." I don't think she gets my level of denial, since it was I who brought up the subject. Once again, I sleep through the treatment, come home, and sleep until 8:30 in the evening.

$3500 SHOT, JULY 22

Yesterday, when Rodriguez said I am doing very well, I told him I want to go to Door County, WI, before my next treatment. He said I should have a neuprin shot to boost my white cells, in other words, my immune system, since I will be traveling and may be exposed to contagion. So today Neena and I return to the Kellogg Cancer Center to get it. The nurse says people think it hurts because it costs so much– $3500. Thank God or the government for Medicare. It will boost my white cells way up over normal. That sounds like leukemia.

We run into Al, Neena's colleague, and his wife Winnie on the way out to the roof parking lot. I have now joined her club. She has cancer in the small bowel, and it has spread to her liver, where surgery caused an infection. Ugh! They are in the process of moving to a condo. She looks okay now, but I feel so badly for her. I had heard that when her cancer was first discovered, it had already spread.

POSTCHEMO, JULY 23, 24

So far, so good. Not queasy like the last time. Hope, hope, hope, but I still feel very weak. Five of my Northwestern students from my spring course come over, which is very sweet of them. Other students whom I don't even know in training programs at Antioch in Seattle and the Art Therapy Institute in Dallas send booklets of get well pictures they made, and students at the Adler Institute in Chicago made me a sort of tree of pictures that Vickie brings.

Later, Sue, Penny, and Margherita come over. Margherita has been so good about visiting. I work on my novel, *Reading Rebecca,* which I haven't been able to do until now.

JULY 25–27

My body is being destroyed. Neuropathy is increasing. I can hardly walk–I'm weak and wobbly. Chemo destroys fast-growing cells like cancer cells, but also hair follicles, thus the hair loss, and the intestinal lining, thus the digestive problems. It also kills nerve cells. The longest ones are those that extend from the spinal cord down the legs and arms, so the first targets of peripheral neuropathy are the feet and fingertips. I don't feel anything very unusual in my fingers except numbness at the ends so that I drop things. My feet are another matter. They feel very strange. The balls of my feet tingle constantly, like when a limb goes to sleep. Ordinarily, after the numbness there is a brief peri-

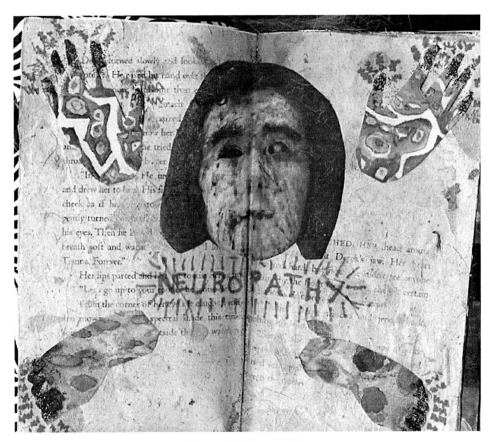

Figure 28. Neuropathy.

od of tingling before all the feeling returns, but in peripheral neuropathy the tingling is constant. Sometimes my feet feel bitter cold and burning hot at the same time. They don't hurt exactly, except occasionally in bed, but the relentless tingling is more than annoying.

My hair is very thin now and big clumps come out in the slightest sweep of my comb. The black tiles of our bathroom floor are carpeted with white hair. My head and the back of my neck are always cold. They miss their soft protection of seventy-eight years. I don't know what to eat. Nothing is appetizing, and I still can't regulate my bowels.

Robinlee comes over with her guitar and we sing out on the deck, which is fun. Former student Susan, whom I haven't seen in years, comes later. Neena and I drive out to the Skokie Lagoons, but I don't get out of the car.

I'm depressed. I feel sunk in a bog of sickness. Going to our vacation house in Door County, WI, seems out of the question. Usually we spend most of the summer there, and we had hoped to have a little time up north between chemo treatments.

Neena's colleague Mary is in town briefly with her new husband, so we are invited to the elegant house of another colleague, Teresa, to see her. When we first arrive, I can barely see due to a visual aura. Everyone is jovial, but I hardly speak. Another guest, Pauline, is talking about all the trips she and Erv are planning around Erv's professional meetings, like Neena and I have done. I don't have that life anymore.

My granddaughter Michaela calls from her Hawaii vacation, which I appreciate, but otherwise I am sunk in depression. More neuropathy. I look it up on the Web, searching for some sort of treatment, but clinical trials have demonstrated nothing that works. Lots of possibilities, but all with hideous side effects. Apparently it gets worse with successive chemos. I'm exhausted. I walk a few paces and have to sit down.

Ellen comes over and that lifts me some. Neena and I go to the Botanic Gardens for the carillon concert, which is lousy. I can hardly walk through the gardens. I'm still depressed.

Sonny calls. His MRI [magnetic resonance imaging] was good. He was worried because he had symptoms that he thought indicated brain tumors. He said you can have brain radiation only once–"only one bite of the apple," as he put it, and he's had it. How terrifying that must be. He had horrible neuropathy with sores on the bottoms of his feet for a year.

JULY 28

I couldn't sleep last night because of leg pain. I finally took some Tylenol® PM and slept a little. I feel somewhat better now, not so sick.

I have lunch at Ruby's Thai restaurant with Neena and her friend Donna, who has had breast cancer three times in the last twenty years. She has the BRCA gene and keeps getting bad odds, but she has refused chemo. She works out a lot to build up her reserves. Should I be doing that? Neena and I take a little walk along the lake. I can't go very far. She waits for me patiently.

I go over my novel *Reading Rebecca,* and Sue comes over. Today is the first day I wear a hat for the sole purpose of covering my balding head.

I call Rodriguez, who says my leg pain isn't neuropathy, it's due to the shot. He wants me to go on a medication because neuropathy has started so early. It will probably get worse.

Neena loses it again—she blows up when I suggest getting some of the clutter out of the back room, which is where we live most of the time. She raves and raves, screaming that she is the only one who does anything for me. She won't lay off me. I feel so helpless. I'm a prisoner, I can't escape. I tell her I want to kill myself. I shouldn't do that, even though it's true. I have no life. My chances are so grim.

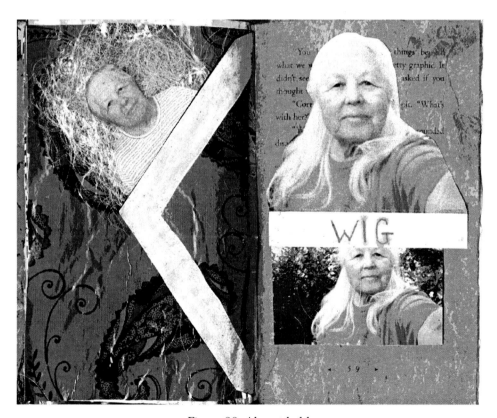

Figure 29. Almost bald.

JULY 29, 30

I drive alone for the first time, to the store. I take a shower standing up for the first time–so the bench comes out of the tub. I'm still tired, and I needed sleeping pills last night. We take a longish walk along the lake.

Elaine, who has had cancer for 10 years, calls and we talk about all her treatments and how she has researched all her needs. It sounds so horrible. She has been in stage IV several years now and was given a death sentence years ago. She will have to be on chemo for the rest of her life. She loves Keith Block, her doctor, and swears by his book (Block, 2009), the one that always leaves me confused and depressed. She tells me that chemo won't be so bad once I am further from surgery. Of course, I am hoping not to need any chemo after this series. I feel depressed from hearing how bad it is for her, but one of her pieces of information is helpful. Aloxi® has prevented nausea for her. I look it up on the Web.

I call Rodriguez's office to ask about Aloxi. Ann tells me that Evanston Hospital doesn't stock it and won't get it. I can have Emend® instead. I hope it works, but I am angry. Why can't I have Aloxi? It helped Elaine, and I don't know if Emend has helped anyone.

I make the mistake of looking over the Block book again. Every time I do so, I get anxious and depressed. I don't know why–maybe because I should be doing more to make myself well. It's still hard to believe I have cancer. The anxiety is physical–a jumpiness in my chest. I have hardly any hair left.

DOOR COUNTY, JULY 31–AUGUST 10

I feel well enough to decide to go to Door County and spend all day packing–I don't know what takes me so long. It almost doesn't seem worth it. I am still feeling anxious and depressed.

Neena does all the driving and all the loading of the car as well. I really appreciate that. I know it's hard for her. I sleep some in the car. Judith and Claire, who have been in the Door house for a week, have it all fixed up and carry in our stuff, make dinner, and do the dishes–very nice of them. They want to talk about cancer too much, and I

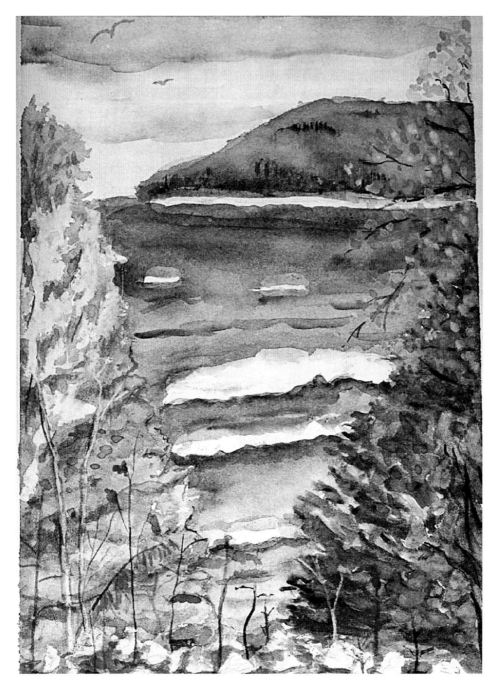

Figure 30. View from Door County window.

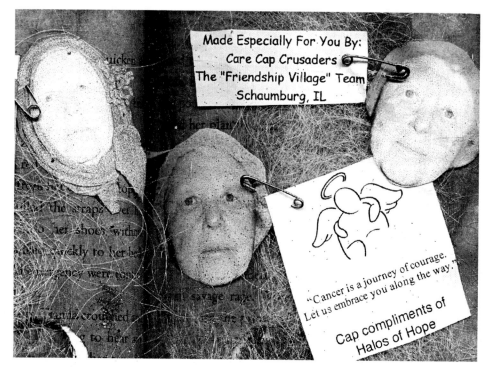

Figure 31. Hats.

have to stop them several times, but they are good friends. They are being very considerate of me. I know cancer scares them (and probably everyone else too). I am still depressed. On May 22, when I had the D&C, I took off my rings and haven't put on jewelry since. Claire notices and states what I am feeling, that I am in mourning.

I walk several trails through the woods, full of wild flowers and butterflies, and I even find a hawk feather. Door County is so renewing. Will I be able to do this next summer? I love summer up here. This whole cancer hell would be even more bitter in winter.

J & C take us to a lovely dinner at the elegant, understated T. Ashwell's restaurant. The food is wonderful and beautifully presented. We eat out on the porch and watch the sun set.

I'm now wearing a hat all the time in front of others. Judith asks me to take it off, but I say no. None of that show-off cue ball look for me. I'm cold most of the time. I hate having my head so vulnerable to the cold and so unsightly with my thin patches of hair. Lucky it isn't winter.

I have been coughing all day. I need to wear a hood so I won't cough. The back of my head and neck get cold. Hats are uncomfortable.

J & C leave. Short hikes. I paint and read a novel, a pleasant change from illness memoirs.

I had diarrhea yesterday and have constipation today. My butt hurts, constant pressure. I go to tai chi at the church nearby. It's held in the parking lot surrounded by fields of lush grasses. It is such a lovely meditation in movement. My feet hurt though. At first I think my shoes are too tight, then I realize it's the neuropathy. Even on a beautiful walk along the limestone layers that edge Lake Michigan at Lynd Point, I think of death. The dread is with me always.

It's the weekend, and Door County is more crowded than I've ever seen it, probably due to the economy—no one is going to Europe. Lisa and Mark have never visited Door County, and for years I have wanted Lisa to see it. Months before I was diagnosed with cancer, she made a reservation at the expensive Country House here. When I was feeling too lousy to think I could make the trip up north myself, Lisa was very gracious about being willing to change plans to visit me in Evanston, even though that would have meant losing their sizeable deposit. Wanting her to see Door County was a strong motivator for my coming.

She and Mark arrive late, and fortunately Lisa loves the Country House. She is picky about mattresses and didn't want to stay at our place. We go to the Sister Bay Bowl, a bowling alley with a restaurant that has the best perch in the world, but we can't get into the dining room so we eat in the noisy smoky bar. Mark likes this real slice of down home Wisconsin, and we all enjoy the perch.

Their first day is cloudy, so I drive Lisa and Mark around for a tour of the northern end of Door. We drop Neena off before going to the Seaquist Orchard Country Store for multiple tastes, which Lisa loves. I'm glad Neena has some time away from us—having other people around can become wearing for her, but later she drives Mark to Peninsula Park to hike. Eric and Keith have been calling me everyday, and she asks me why my kids call me so often. They call at home too, but in our larger house there, she is not so aware of the calls. I tell her it's because they love me and are concerned about me and that I appreciate it. I think she gets annoyed with them because she wishes that they would do more than call, that they would help out in some way.

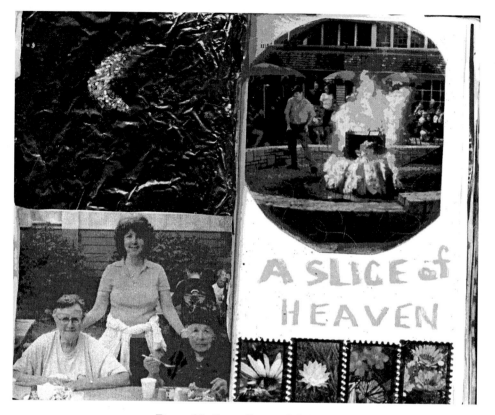

Figure 32. Door County fish boil.

Mark takes a nap back at the Country House, and Lisa and I sit out in the garden and have the most frank talk about sex ever. We have an elegant dinner at T. Ashwell's, which Lisa says is some of the best food she's ever had. The next day, she and I go to the lovely Edgewood Orchard gallery, where we sit in the sculpture garden and talk some more, this time about Mark's son Gabriel, whom she is helping him raise. In the evening we all go to a fish boil held outside the Viking restaurant, where we eat outside, and Lisa and Mark are suitably impressed by the flames shooting high above the restaurant. That's followed by a great sunset at the dock. I am really glad to be able to spend time with Lisa in Door County. She and Mark want to return. I feel good that I am able to drive almost halfway home from Door County.

When I get home, I call my brother: "How are you, Sonny?"

"Tickety-boo and jake-a-loo."

"And your scans?"

"Great. I'm the luckiest guy alive. Harriet says I'll live forever."

"I'm Harriet."

"I mean Joan." That's his wife. He never could keep us straight. What would Freud say?

"When do you have to get your next scan?"

"Well, because of the inoperable growth near my spine, I have to get them every three months. It's grown, but the doc says there's room for growth."

"Do you ever worry about all that radiation?"

"When you've had your head bolted down for the gamma knife, a couple more rads don't make much difference. My doctor says there's a new chemo for renal cancer given by injection without side effects that I'll get if I need it, but I don't now."

There's no whining in this guy's presence. How does he do it?

ROUGH RIDE, CHEMO #3, AUGUST 11

I'm waiting in the examining room for Rodriguez when a resident, a heavy dark-skinned young woman from another country, comes in. Do I have any questions? I ask her about Emend that I am supposed to get for nausea. She says it is an appetite stimulant. Nurse Ann comes in and says no but adds that I need the shot to raise my white blood cell count again. I say no. She says I had it before so I have to have it each time because my white cell count is low. I say no, it was because I was traveling with a suppressed immune system and could have picked up some wayward bug. I'm not going to travel now. She goes out to check and comes back with an apology. This sort of carelessness is upsetting. Rodriguez comes in and says no to the Emend appetite stimulant question. He gets me a printout to prove it. They seem annoyed with the resident, who is speaking heresy to a patient. Two out of two errors—that doesn't instill confidence.

When Rodriguez does a pelvic, I make the mistake of asking him what he is looking for. Before, I had thought he was monitoring my healing from the surgery, but why would he have to do that now? He says he is checking for tumors in the pelvic floor and abdomen this kind of cancer can spawn. Something else for me to dread.

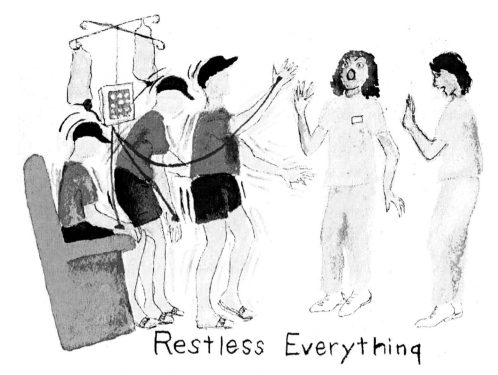

Figure 33. Restless everything.

I have a long wait in the Kellogg Cancer Center because Rod-riguez hasn't signed the chemo order. Another flub? After it eventual-ly gets going, I am partially knocked out, but awake enough to know I have restless legs. I can't stop moving them. Then I get restless every-thing else and keep jumping up out of my chair, sitting in another chair, jumping up, and coming back to the first one. A couple of nurs-es are yelling at me to stay still because I will interfere with the chemo flow. I don't even answer them. Next I wake up in a hospital bed. I don't remember being moved. I keep trying to push down the sides so I can escape.

Neena had stayed with me during all the hours of my previous chemo sessions, but since I slept through them, this time after getting me settled she has gone to her office at Northwestern. When she returns she can't find me and no one she asks knows where I am. Eventually she locates me in the room with the bed. Later she tells me I kept asking to go to the bathroom every fifteen minutes. In the bed my legs looked as though I was running, she says. When they finally unhook me, the nurse says I have been there an extra hour because my moving compressed the chemo infusion tube.

An aide pushes me in a wheelchair the long way to the parking lot, and I want to tip him, but I can't find my wallet. I insist that we go back. The bag I had brought had been left in the first room before I was moved to the one with a bed, but my wallet isn't there either. We go back to the parking lot, and I ask Neena to tip the aide. Later, I find my wallet at home. I had not brought it with me. I never do. My brain was far too fogged to put any of that together at the time. It's 5 PM and I crash. I sleep until 5 AM.

POSTCHEMO, AUGUST 12–21

Hooray, no sick feeling the first couple days. Emend works. Then the sick-to-my-stomach feeling returns and stays for two weeks. I'm weak and easily fatigued too.

Neena's department has a picnic on the lakefront. I spend most of it talking to Winnie. She looks wasted from her cancer, very thin. She says she can't gain weight. She has had cancer for two years. It is an unusual kind of the small intestine with no special treatment for it, so she is getting colon cancer treatment. She says her cancer is incurable, that her treatment is palliative. She'll resume chemo after she and Al move to their new condo, which they are doing so Al won't have to deal with the house. She's already planning for her death. In the condo, she won't be able to dye fabric for the wall hangings she makes. We talk about death. She says everyone has to die sometime. I want to talk to her about it more, but Neena motions to me for us to leave. Maybe I'll call Winnie and get together with her after she's moved.

We go to another picnic, this one indoors because it has started to rain. People are glad I could come. They seem surprised. I look for an empty chair because I have to sit down.

The rain clears and several days later we have a beautiful day for the Cancer Wellness Center meditation at the Botanic Garden. Someone wearing a large straw hat looks like Claudia, but I'm not sure it's her. Everyone is meditating when we arrive, so I can't talk to her. I decide that the woman isn't her because her hands look like a suburban matron's. Afterwards, she talks to us, and indeed it is her. She wants me to make art with her. I suppose I am being added to her list of friends lined up to do things for her. On the drive home Neena is totally tense, shaking her hands. So much for the calming effects of meditation and the gardens.

August 20 is a horrible, horrible day. I decide to work on the CD of the artwork that will accompany the art therapy book because it doesn't look as though Tony is able to do it since he doesn't have Photoshop. I work to exhaustion on the color enhancement, cropping, captioning, and numbering for almost 200 pictures. As I am titling the chapter picture folders, I discover there is NO CHAPTER 17! That means renumbering the pictures of Chapters 18 to 27 and changing their text references. I am exhausted. There is no way. The chapter numbering must have gotten mixed up when Isabel, the editor, and I were going back and forth arranging the different sections, which meant changing chapter numbers. I think that was around the time I was getting tests for cancer. How else could I have made such a careless mistake?

The only solution other than renumbering the pictures and the text references is to create a Chapter 17. I resurrect one from the first edition that I had eliminated, edit it, and take out the pictures because I no longer have access to them. I use pictures from other portions of the book. Then I have problems burning the CD. The whole thing is an exhausting nightmare. I have to get out of the house, so Neena and I go out to dinner–tapas.

THE LIGHT OF DAY, AUGUST 22

The Off Campus Writers Workshop (OCWW) newsletter announcing its fall speaker schedule arrives. Patricia Lear will be speaking on memoirs from devastating illnesses. How serendipitous for me. This is a talk I have to hear. She will also critique fifteen pages of the first ten manuscripts sent to her. The opportunity for a critique of my writing is enticing, but I have not even been able to look at what I have written here. Forcing myself to write about what I am going through has been hard. Mostly I keep putting it off, and I have not wanted to go back and read it, much less do any editing. Nor have I read any portion of this journal to Neena or to anyone else. Do I want others to see such personal revelations?

I plunge ahead because how often would the topic of memoir writing about the impact of a major illness be available to me? I tackle editing the first fifteen pages, all of it before any treatment began, and deliver the packet right away. Since the speaker will review only the first ten manuscripts sent to her, I don't even take a chance on the mail. She lives only about fifteen minutes from me, so I drive to her apartment and put the manuscript directly into her mailbox. Only after I drop it off do I consider that my work might be read aloud at the meeting. In my haste to be among the first ten, I haven't even given this possibility a thought. I feel as though I am closing my eyes, taking a breath, and stepping off the end of a high diving board into insubstantial air. The speaker is scheduled for two days after my last

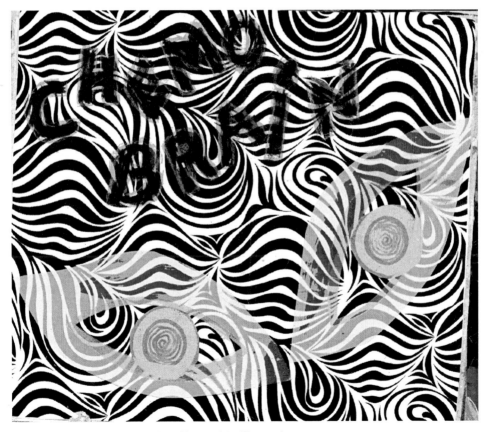

Figure 34. Chemo brain.

chemo, almost two months from now, so maybe I won't even feel well enough to go to the meeting. I'm not sure I want all this dark stuff to see the light of day.

TAKING STOCK

Chemo reactions: Strange when washing in the shower, no pubic hair–like a child. My nails are harder than ever and long. I trim them so I can type without messing up, but I keep fumbling and dropping things. It's the neuropathy, not just long nails. My feet feel funny too. Sometimes there is fatigue, panting, and rapid heart beats just from walking up the stairs, and dizzy, woozy feelings, even during the good times. My head and the back of my neck are always cold. I wear a knit cap all the time now, even in bed.

Chemo brain: things fall out of my head. Example: I asked Neena if she wanted some more of the soup I had made. She said yes, but I never got up to fill her empty bowl. I simply forgot as soon as I had asked her.

What to do? Only one thing, turn this nightmare into a work of art.

MEDIEVAL TORTURE, AUGUST 24

I go to the hospital to see the oncology radiologist, a very nice Indian woman with a ready smile. She does a pelvic and examines my breasts. No tumors. I've healed well from the surgery, she says. My uterine tumor was small, only a little more than two centimeters. The radiology, she says, is for the local area because tumors are likely to form there.

She describes the radiation process in grisly detail. I will be placed on a cart, in stirrups, examined and washed with antiseptic. Things will be stuffed in every lower orifice, a Foley catheter in my bladder and something in my rectum. I think these are for X-rays. The cart will be wheeled to the X-ray room to shoot pictures, then I'll be wheeled to a treatment room. A plastic "tampon" will be stuck up my vagina and placed with careful measurements. A wire will be inserted in it and a radioactive "seed" shot into me by a machine. The contraption will move up and down inside me for half an hour in the area to be radiated. No one will be in the room with me because I will be radio-active. The whole process will take an hour. She warns me that I have to defecate before coming in because a full bowel will push everything out of position. With all my constipation problems, I'll have to get up at some ungodly hour to poop before I get there at nine.

I will need three treatments at weekly intervals, starting in three weeks. After the first one I won't need more X-rays, so those will take less time. I ask about side effects. She says the catheter might cause a bladder infection. At home, I read the written material she has given me. The x-ray can burn my vagina. The procedure can cause cramping and nausea. It's bad enough that I am allowing myself to be poisoned, how can I go willingly into this medical torture chamber?

From the hospital we go to the Botanic Gardens. The day is beautiful and the gardens gorgeous, but I just keep thinking of the torture. We have supper on the terrace overlooking the water and a bank of brilliant yellow blossoms. I don't like what I've ordered, so I get another entrée. Grilled salmon. It's delicious. I think I'm compensating for all my fear and sorrow. We go to the carillon concert, which isn't very good. Sue and Al meet us there. Sometimes Sue makes jokes about my condition. I don't know whether to laugh or cry.

At home, Neena says something about the radiation being good because I will get it over with.

I snap, "You're not the one who has to have it."

Neena says, "I hate to see you so sad."

I say, "I'm being tortured."

"No, you're being treated."

"It doesn't feel like a treat to me." This is the medical maw that will chew me up. The crazy part is that I will allow them to do this to me. I will authorize my insurance to pay them to torture me. I feel so helpless. I imagine myself with my legs spread apart, totally vulnerable as they stuff instruments into me.

DOOR COUNTY, AUGUST 26–30

Neena does all the driving and I doze some. The long drive must tire her. It rains until we hit the Wisconsin border, then the sun comes out. Welcome to farmland. It's good to be here. Tai chi, Sentinel Trail at Peninsula State Park, butterfly walk at Newport Park with a naturalist, and the Monarch Trail. Caterpillars and chrysalises that are translucent so that I can see the wings–fascinating.

Sue and Al were supposed to visit, but Sue calls from a hospital saying she may have had a heart attack, but the tests show nothing. She thinks it's a virus and she wants to come the next day, but I have to tell her not to, that I can't be near her because she might be contagious. I feel really badly about telling her this, but I am being careful with my compromised immune system. I am going to cancel theater and opera tickets in the fall.

Fall comes to Door County in a burst of rain and wind, dark clouds, and spots of turning leaves. We decide to go home a day early. We have breakfast at the Viking restaurant and leave Door County on a beautiful clear windy day. We stop at Cave Point, and I walk along the bluff of the rocky shore and watch the waves pound the limestone shelves.

DAY BEFORE CHEMO, AUGUST 31

I finish reading *Between Me and the River* by Carrie Host (2006). I'm not sure what I think about it. She went through cancer hell, but she describes a perfect family–a dream of a husband, kids who are never bratty, a mother and sisters who come to take care of her. Do I believe her? The difficulty in writing a memoir is being open and honest without hurting anyone.

Neena is scheduled to see her doctor the day of my first radiation just when it is supposed to be finished. She wants to keep her appointment and leave me in a hospital waiting room for an hour after having instruments stuffed up me and being irradiated. She gives me a hard time about changing her appointment. I slump into a depression, comparing Neena with Carrie Host's husband, who couldn't do enough for her and was always loving, she writes, although I don't say anything about the book to Neena. She agrees to change the appointment. I am very grateful.

One of the reasons for coming home from Door County a day early was to finish Chapter 17 of the art therapy book. I still can't open Tony's attachment of references for it. Finally I finish it anyway. I walk around the block, but my left hip hurts. I hope my hip replacement isn't coming apart.

NEEDLED IN CHEMO #4, SEPTEMBER 1

Chemo brain keeps thinking this is chemo number three, rather than number four. Another resident comes into the examining room before Rodriguez again. She asks if I have questions and tells me the horrible side effects of radiation. Rodriguez comes in and talks about risk/benefits of radiation. He doesn't like to talk about side effects.

"If you look up aspirin," he says, "you'll see three pages of side effects. If there is high risk, we would discuss it with you." He examines me and apologizes as usual. I like that. "Everything looks fine," he pronounces.

Upstairs in the Cancer Center, the chemo nurse can't get the infusion needle in. She calls in someone else. I get stuck several times. After a while, they check it and say it isn't working so they take the needle out. I have to wait an hour for a needle expert. She sticks it in the other hand. I have become a human pin cushion, getting stuck each time for blood draws as well as multiple sticks for the chemo. My veins seem to have vanished.

Almost as soon as the drip gets going, a young, energetic-looking woman comes in announcing, "I am Heather, the music therapist. What would you like to do?"

"I'd like to be entertained and have fun." No soul-searching therapy for me.

Heather goes to get her guitar and keyboard. She hands me a songbook and we sing together, *Sittin' by the Dock of the Bay.* I make up chemo words for it and then we sing *Blowin' in the Wind.* She writes down my words, and we sing them together. It's fun.

"I'll type up your lyrics," she says, "and send them to you." Here they are:

Sittin' in My La-Z-Boy
(Melody: [*Sittin' on*] *The Dock of the Bay* by Otis Redding)

Sittin' in my La-Z-Boy
Just waitin' for the chemo to drip,
Watchin' all the nurses go by.
This ain't my idea of a trip.
Yeah, I'm sittin' in the Kellogg Center,

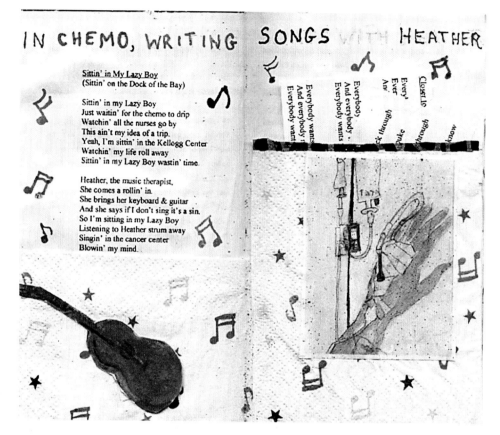

Figure 35. Music therapy.

Watchin' my life roll away,
Sittin' in my La-Z-Boy wastin' time.

Heather, the music therapist,
She comes a rollin' in.
She brings her keyboard and guitar,
And says if I don't sing it's a sin.
So I'm sittin' in my La-Z-Boy,
Listenin' to Heather strum away.
Singin' in the Cancer Center,
Blowin' my mind.

A Mystery I Don't Know
(Melody: *Blowin' in the Wind* by Bob Dylan)

How many drips must the chemo tick through
Before the cancer cells die?
How many times must I feel like I'll puke
Before I can stop asking why?
How many times must the poison blast through
Before I will finally cry?

The answer, my friend, is a mystery I don't know,
The answer is a mystery I don't know.

Not exactly upbeat, but the words are spontaneous and capture how I am feeling.

The good news is that after our songfest, hydroxyzine knocks me out and doesn't cause restlessness as the Benadryl did. At home I crash at six and don't get up until 8:30 the next morning.

AFTER CHEMO, SEPTEMBER 2–10

I feel better than I ever have on the day after chemo. I have a normal appetite, and although a bit woozy, wobbly, and dizzy, I don't have that sick feeling. I take two walks, one along the lake. I finish Chapter 17 of my art therapy book and send it and the CD to Isabel. Hooray! What a load off my back (Wadeson, 2010).

Lots of visitors, which is a good distraction because I start feeling yucky after a couple days. Feeling worse and worse. Ten days after chemo I still feel nauseous. This is the longest stretch yet. Ann says it may be due to dehydration, but I am bloating myself with water as it is.

ALTERED BOOK

I go to an Altered Book workshop at the Cancer Wellness Center anyway. I've never made an altered book before, and the project interests me. The teacher, Janie Baskin, says we can do a book on the seasons or travel, or several other topics she mentions, but I say no, I am going to make a cancer book. Cancer isn't on her long list of topics.

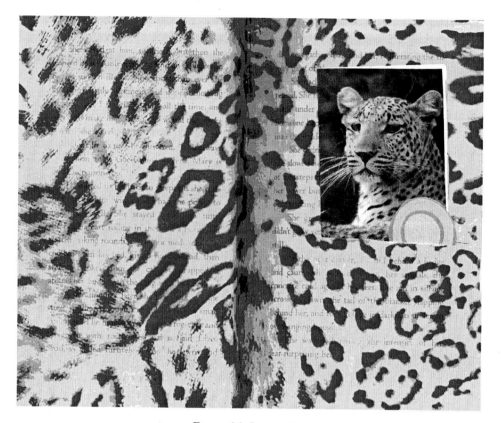

Figure 36. Leopards.

Janie has brought a number of books from which we can select to alter. I am attracted to a blue book with a picture of a young woman with black hair on the front. It's a strange choice because I will probably glue some other image on the cover to suit my subject. For the moment, however, I like the young woman. While we are looking through the books and the papers, pictures, ribbons, and other materials Janie has brought, one of the other women in the class tells me she still has restless feet problems from Taxol three years after treatment. Scarey.

Janie has also brought some altered books she has made that have intriguing pockets, peep holes, coverings on pages, and objects hanging from them. She instructs us to tear out lots of pages throughout our book, because otherwise it will become too bulky with all we glue into it. She teaches us to make slanted pockets. I peruse the papers she has brought and bypass the flowery ones for a camouflage pattern. After completing the pocket, I look over pictures she has brought for something to put in it and select one that looks like Hamlet holding Yoric's skull. I hadn't intended to portray death, but that's what emerges. Hidden death, tucked away in a pocket (see Figure 17, Death, p. 42).

Janie shows us how to make another kind of pocket, and for this one I choose a leopard skin pattern. There isn't time to find anything to put into it, but at home I find some leopards that I develop into a booklet of images of strength. So here I am, starting out with death and strength. I guess that fits my current state of mind.

The death picture needs something else, so I scan a painting I've made of birds on the beach, reduce it on the printer, and glue on the reduced image. I seem to be adding some life to the death image. I become totally absorbed in working on my altered book most of the day and end up exhausted. I feel so horrible I have to cancel my appointment with the oncology nutritionist.

SEPTEMBER 11

Claudia has asked me about doing art with her, and we had set it up for today. She doesn't show up, so I call her. She forgot and made a breakfast date, but she comes over afterwards. I suggest a warm-up picture, and she finds significant meaning in it. Then I do a guided imagery for her, calling up her various strengths and resources. She gets into it. She is convinced that she is in denial, but says she expects to get recurrences and more treatment. She isn't getting sick from chemo the way I am, which she attributes to acupuncture. She is surprised when I tell her I haven't cried. I get depressed, I say. She doesn't. She is planning to visit her mother next week to tell her she has cancer. I feel glad I don't have to do that. As we finish up, she says she is going to buy some art materials, so I guess she thinks the session has been helpful. Only after she gets out the door does she remember to thank me. Although I hadn't intended this as therapy, essentially it was–two hours worth for free–with art supplies thrown in. I suppose I have been drafted into her cadre of helpers.

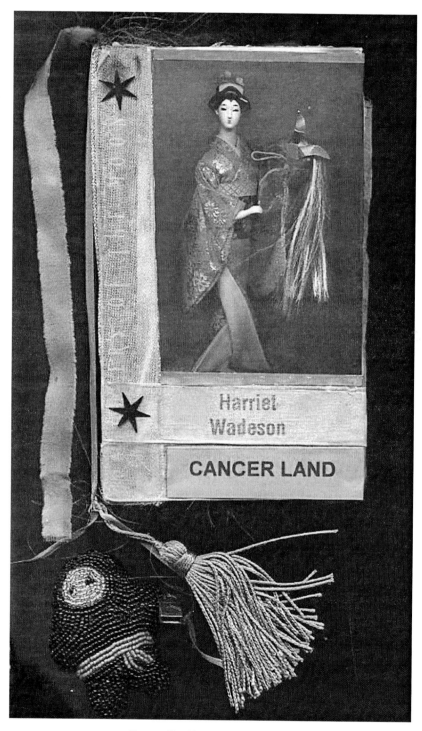

Figure 37. Altered book cover.

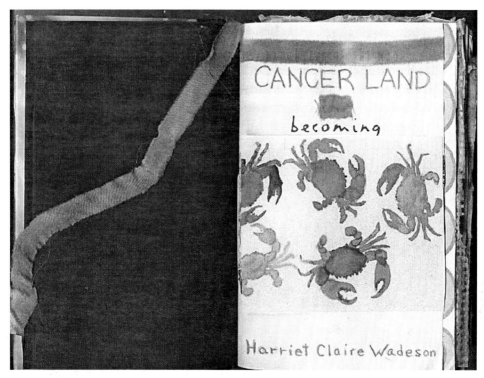

Figure 38. Cancer Land title page.

SEPTEMBER 12, 13

I am feeling better, but I'm still weak and tired. I go to the Farmers Market, the Saturday tasting at Schaefer's wine shop, and in the evening the potluck at Alice's. We drive there with Judith and Claire. Since Alice lives far from others in Hyde Park, it's a small group, which is nice because we can all talk together, although I am interrupted several times, making me feel as though I don't exist.

I have a better attitude toward radiation tomorrow. Instead of dread, I'll just get it over–an hour out of my life. I work on the altered book, pasting ribbons on the front to cover the original title and author. I name the book *Cancer Land.* That feels right to me. I put crabs on the title page. I go out and take a walk by the lake. I make ratatouille and eat only vegetables so I can poop tomorrow before radiation, as ordered by the radiologist.

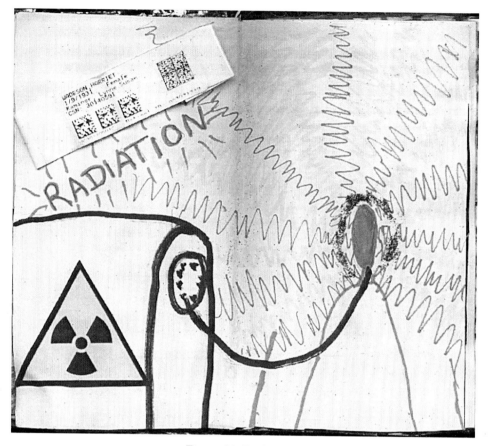

Figure 39. Radiation.

RADIATION, SEPTEMBER 14

I get up early to prep, mainly to poop, which I do. I feel woozy from premedication. The radiologist, who had seemed so nice when I saw her before, is very rough with the insertions. Fortunately, she doesn't have to stick something in my rectum, but she inserts the catheter in my bladder and pushes the pod for the wire (which she refers to as a tampon, but it is ten times larger than any tampon) into the top of my vagina. It is held in place with tape all over my bottom. I am slid onto various carts and tables as I am moved from the examining room to the X-ray room to the radioactive treatment room. All the rooms are freezing. I have to wait about an hour alone in the treatment room for all the calculations to be made, while lying still so as not to dislodge all the apparatus inside me. I doze and listen to my i-Pod. Finally, a technician comes in and inserts a wire into the pod that is in me and leaves. The machine beeps for the half hour of the radiation. The whole process is barbaric. Particularly unnerving is the rough handling by the radiologist who was deceptively sweet and friendly initially.

I will drink cranberry juice so I won't get a bladder infection from the catheter. At home I crash and even fall asleep at the computer.

SEPTEMBER 15

Last winter, Robinlee and I submitted a proposal to the American Art Therapy Association (AATA) to present a paper describing our community mural project for the Three Crowns Retirement Park at the annual conference in Dallas in November, more than a month after I will finish chemo. Feeling almost normal, I reserve the airline ticket. When I am not sick to my stomach, I can plan. This is the first time I have felt able to make a commitment to a future obligation.

I work on the altered book. Some paper I've taken home from the workshop reminds me of cells, so I use it for introductory pages about my Pap test showing suspicious cells. It's fun to find materials that fit my experience so well.

I go to a meditation group at Evanston Hospital and like it, especially the leader David. When I introduce myself, he says I am not just an art therapist, I am an eminent one. He knows that I have written books on art therapy. I wonder how.

I go to the second session of the altered books workshop. Janie Baskin, the teacher, is impressed with what I have done, the two pockets, the cover, a title page with crabs, and the beginning pages about my Pap test. Books the others are working on are cutsie.

SEPTEMBER 16, 17

I work more on the altered book. I have moved to the ending. I want to focus on what life will be like after I have left this chemo hell, making pictures of going to the theater and concerts, traveling, spending time outdoors and with my family. I use colored papers and pho-

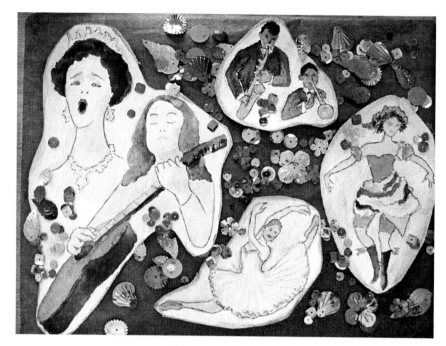

Figure 40. Concerts.

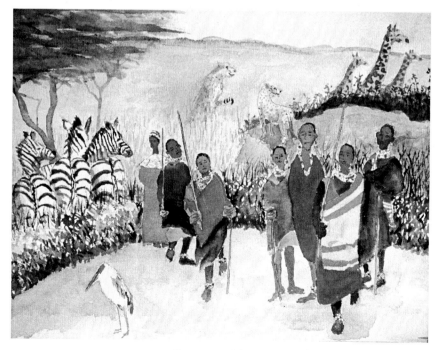

Figure 41. Africa.

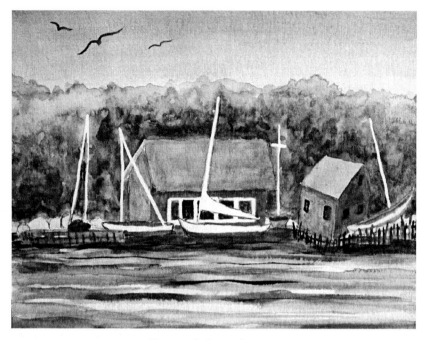

Figure 42. Door County.

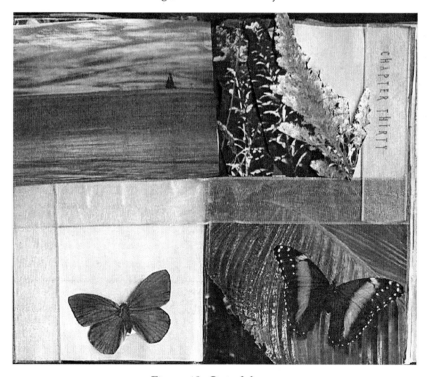

Figure 43. Out of doors.

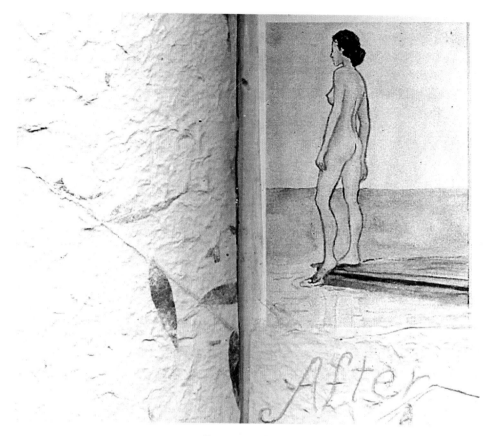

Figure 44. After.

tos of Neena, my brother, children, and grandchildren. I sprinkle on glitter. I depict travel with paintings I have made of Africa and Door County. I paint dancers and musicians and surround them with sequins. I enjoy making these.

I introduce this section with a painting of a young woman dipping her toe in the water and gazing out over it. I particularly like this picture. It has a delicacy about it. The woman looks tentative. I don't expect my body to look like hers again, but I hope one day that I will feel good about it, that it will be healthy and trustworthy to me once more. I get lost in my book.

I go to lunch with Margherita at Ala Carte, a take-out place with good food and a few tables. She has been so consistent in staying in touch. She brings books of her Italian grandfather's sculptures, which are lovely. She has been telling me of the family travails in trying to divide them up. We go to the lighthouse and sit in the sun overlooking the beach. The area around the magnificent old mansion next to the lighthouse, now art center, is very nice. There's even a small waterfall I'd never seen designed by famous landscape architect Jens Jenson.

Chaya Sara calls because I am supposed to see her for a wig trim, but her child is sick. She had invited us for *Rosh Hashanah* dinner tomorrow, but now that has to be canceled too. I appreciate her realizing that I am trying to avoid any contagion, but disappointed to miss Rosh Hashanah. She says she called her friend Faygie, whom we had met at her house, and Faygie wants to invite us.

ROSH HASHANAH, SEPTEMBER 18

Neena and I arrive at Faygie's in time to light the Sabbath candles at sundown, but you'd never know a big dinner was planned. The large table in the living room isn't set and no one seems to be around. Eventually we light candles with Faygie's daughter who shows us how to say the prayer. We want to help with dinner, but are told there is nothing to do. Faygie is busy in the kitchen—she has a catering business. I talk a little with her daughter and husband, both of whom are nice, but mostly we just sit and wait for almost four hours. Faygie comes in at one point and in response to Neena's question, tells us the long, long story of her entry into this community in a tale that goes from Israel to Holland to India to Cleveland. In the end, we tell her she should write about her odyssey. Who would ever suspect this orthodox Jewish mother of eight of having been a globe-trotting hippie?

The food is good and there is plenty of it. Throughout the dinner Faygie gives us lessons in Judaism. A bunch of young girls from the community's school—out-of-towners with no place to go for the holiday—joins us. I am amazed at their conversation—whether it is permissible to ride a bike on *Shabbat*. This is the concern of adolescent girls who have clearly given attention to their hair and clothes? The family is very nice and certainly gracious in hosting us. This is such a strange new/old world for me.

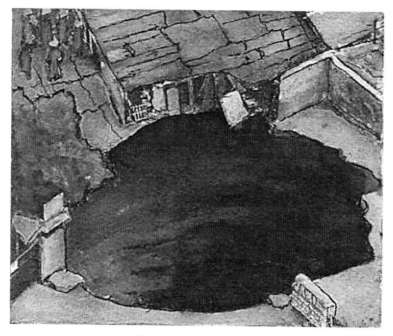

Figure 45. Black hole.

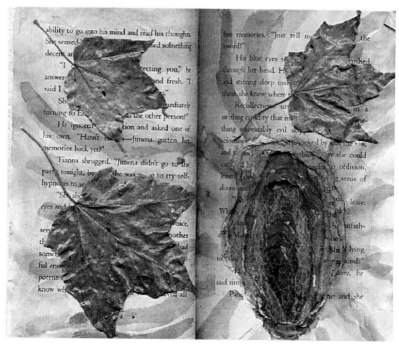

Figure 46. Black hole dug in the book.

SEPTEMBER 19, 20

I go to the Farmers Market and work more on the altered book. It is consuming me. I paint a black hole inspired by a sink hole I see in a magazine and begin digging a hole through many pages, the black hole into which my life has fallen. I have collected some autumn leaves that I shellac and glue on to look as though they are being sucked into the hole.

I take Neena to the lighthouse, surprised that despite her thirty years in Evanston, she has never been there. She is enchanted. We walk on the beach, the grounds of the mansion, and the park next to it.

We go to the Botanic Gardens—wonderful. I walk more than I have in a long time. My hip doesn't hurt. Hooray. I put a pad in my shoe since one leg is longer than the other due to my hip replacement. Jeanne comes over and brings soup, a cake she made, and tomatoes. We have a nice visit.

RADIATION #2, SEPTEMBER 21

The radiologist is rough again in stuffing in the huge "tampon," which is so much larger than any Tampax! I tell her to stop messing around with the front when she has to put it in the vagina. Then after being slid from the table for the insertion to a cart to a table for the X-rays in another room to a cart again to a table in the treatment room, I am left lying there for half an hour while the radiologist works on another patient. Once again, I have to lie still in a freezing room with all the stuff stuck in me. Then half an hour of radiation while the machine beeps. I remain still. I listen to my i-Pod throughout. I tell the radiologist that next week I will likely not feel well because I'll have chemo prior to the radiation, so I don't want to have to wait.

CHEMO #5, SEPTEMBER 22

Rodriguez is very positive—one more treatment after today and then no more after the CAT scan, then scans once or twice a year. I get a different poison today because of neuropathy—Taxotre. It is like Taxol but is not supposed to have the same neuropathy effects. No

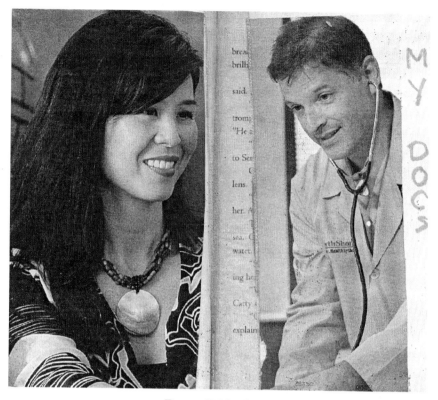

Figure 47. My docs.

knock-out meds this time. Colleen the nutritionist and Heather the music therapist come. I write another song and sing the old ones. Taxotre doesn't take as long to drip in, so I get off early.

SEPTEMBER 23, 24

So far so good, I'm not nauseous, but I am wobbly from the scopolamine patch that is supposed to prevent nausea. I see Dr. Mendoza-Temple, the integrative medicine doc. I like her, and she sure is prettier than Block, who is also an integrative medicine doc. She recommends supplements, so I spend $110 for a stash.

ACUPUNCTURE, SEPTEMBER 25

I try out acupuncture at Highland Park Hospital with Molly. I like her but I don't know if it does any good. Neena and I have a nice lunch afterwards in Highland Park. In the evening, we go to a staged reading at Northwestern in a small theatre. I wear a protective mask. It is my first theatre experience since starting chemo. We leave at intermission. I am still not taking chances on catching something because of my suppressed immune system. I've already given away my ticket to the first of the Goodman Theatre series.

SEPTEMBER 26, 27

I feel rotten even though the pharmacist at the hospital said they've pulled out the big guns for me to fight nausea. It takes me all morning to get downstairs. Mostly I just sit and stare. I have diarrhea (I was constipated) and spend most of the day on the toilet. Where does it all

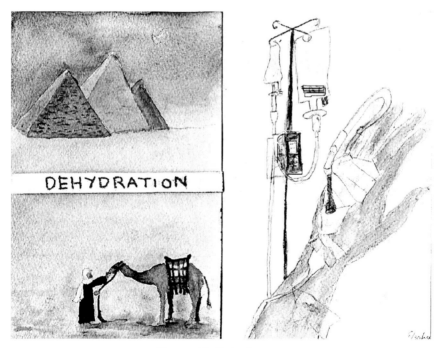

Figure 48. Dehydration.

come from? I am eating very little. I have back aches too. I can't do anything. Could acupuncture have done this?

Deb comes over with soup and gifts from her trip to Costa Rica. Neena and I drive to the lake, but I can hardly walk—I'm dizzy, nauseous, and my legs and fingers don't work.

LAST RADIATION, SEPTEMBER 28

I feel dizzy and unbalanced with diarrhea, so I ask the radiologist not to leave me waiting on the table and to be more gentle in inserting the tube. So it's not as bad as before. I go to Whole Foods to buy cranberry juice because she says I can still get a bladder infection.

HYDRATION, SEPTEMBER 29

Today is my mother's 106th birthday. What would she think if she saw how miserable I am? Maybe Lisa has taken her place—she gets upset when I feel lousy.

I cancel my massage appointment because I am being sent to the hospital to be rehydrated due to my nonstop diarrhea dehydration. My bottom is sore from all the activity. Fortunately, my electrolytes are okay so I don't need several hours more of drips for them. So it's back to the Kellogg Cancer Center yet again. Once more I get multiple sticks for the saline solution drip—the usual trouble finding a vein.

SEPTEMBER 30, OCTOBER 1

The hydration hasn't helped me to feel any better, so I have to have another one. I get stuck four times. I still have diarrhea and can't sleep because my bottom hurts from it.

I go to the Indian restaurant with Margherita, but the food doesn't taste good to me. I can hardly walk I am so dizzy—weaving all over the place—so I take off the scopolamine patch I've been wearing for nausea because it affects balance.

I give away our *Tosca* tickets, the first of our Lyric Opera series.

OCTOBER 2

I took one Imodium® pill two days ago, so now I am constipated. Elaine visits and brings her lunch. She is in her tenth year of cancer and is on chemo permanently. I have been depressed since, I'm not sure why. Maybe because I am constipated. Maybe because hearing her challenges all my denial. I can eat hardly any dinner.

We were planning to drive to Door County tomorrow. Sue and Al are going to our house there today and I had hoped to spend time with them in Door County. I can see no way I can make it. Letting go of that plan to go tomorrow is a relief. I do want to see the fall color, but the forecast is for rain. Maybe in a few days. . . . All of this is wearing me down.

OCTOBER 3

My butt hurts because I am so constipated. I'm weak and I can't do anything. Sue calls and says it's cold and rainy in Door County. The forecast is for rain all week, so I decide not to go at all. I spend the whole day lying down or sitting on the toilet. Neena keeps telling me not to be depressed. If I stand up and I walk from one room to another, I have to lie down again. I can't eat.

Not until 2 PM do I realize today is Keith's birthday. Keith's line has been busy twice. I'm not going to talk, I'll just wish him happy birthday.

I'm more depressed than any day so far. The anniversary of delivering him myself in an ambulance two months premature may be the reason. Remembering Keith's birthday seems to pull it all together. I'm reminded of the abortion I had at this time of year, discovering myself pregnant shortly after my husband left, just lying on the couch watching the day slide into evening. Keith was born forty-eight years ago. The abortion was thirty-eight years ago. I am damaged. Recently, Keith visited the Bethesda Carderock Springs house where we all used to live—he and Lisa have been talking to me about it. It has been improved and is assessed at $1 million. I was swindled into selling it cheap. I don't want to think about that. Now, like then, my body is damaged.

Neena says I'll get better. I'm glad she thinks so. My cancer is hard on her and she has trouble caring for me. In addition to atrial fibrillation and arthritis, she needs surgery for a cataract, but she can't get it while I am sick. My neuropathy is worse. If I get better, I will need to make a plan. A plan for what to do if I have a recurrence. Neena won't be able to care for me. I might have to move to some sort of care facility. Or end it.

SUKKOTH, OCTOBER 4

I stop typing this journal. I have tried to stay current, typing my handwritten scrawls into my computer soon after writing them, but I can't do it anymore. It's all I can do to scribble something into my notebook every few days. (I am typing this part six months later.)

I feel a little better, although I am still weak. We go to *Sukkoth* at Faygie's–a cross-cultural experience of about thirty or forty people. They have built a hut in the back yard, and all the men sit together at the center of the horseshoe the tables form with the women and kids along the sides. Faygie treats us as special, introducing us as dear friends, and she explains all the ritual stuff to us. Tons of food are set out, but I don't like any of it, so I eat very little. I don't like anything these days. The men sing in an old Jewish style and argue, in what I guess is the Talmudic tradition, about trivia. There are several know-it-alls–one who is particularly arrogant.

I had never been to a *Sukkoth* before. This one is like going back in time to some other era in some other place. Back in the house, Faygie shows me her art. Where she finds the time amidst eight children and all that cooking, I don't know. It is so kind of her to include us in this ancient traditional harvest celebration among her very large family and many friends.

OCTOBER 5

I feel better, not as depressed. Neena and I go to the Botanic Gardens. Gorgeous day with chrysanthemums all in bloom, but I can hardly walk. I am exhausted after every few steps. So I do a lot of sitting. We take a shuttle to the new science building, but don't go in because I can't walk around. Later, Sue stops by with goodies from Door. I finally poop—now I am constipated again, and I still can't eat.

OCTOBER 6

Hooray, I poop several times. This preoccupation with my toilet problems that has been going on for months now is an intrusion in my life I never knew before. Will I ever be free from this again?

It's cold and rainy. Fall is here. I have some energy and take care of a lot of stuff. I go to meditation at the hospital, part of their cancer wellness program. The meditation is very soothing. A woman cries and I tell her I feel badly for her. She comes over to my chair and hugs me. I am surprised the leader doesn't offer her support.

I eat steak and half a baked potato, the first time for normal protein.

HOMES FOR THE ELDERLY, OCTOBER 7

Animals sneak off to the woods to die. Where do old people go to spend their last days? They used to be cared for in the bosoms of their families, but rarely are these days. Some die quickly and save their families wear and care. Others are warehoused in nursing homes. Some, like many of the older women in my Aqua Fitness group, plan to go to a life-care facility while they are still able to make the move. The concept here is "gracious living," to live independently in your own apartment while receiving services such as restaurants, transportation, and lively activities. Then to "graduate" (or whatever the opposite of graduation is) to assisted living and then nursing care, all within the same facility.

For the past five years, Neena has been complaining that our house is too much for us and that we should move to a condo. I have maintained that if we are going to all the trouble of a move, we should move to a life-care facility, like the "Splashers," as we call ourselves in my aqua group. Finding the right place involves a long looking and researching process, so I began several years ago. I looked into Westminster Place, where both of us had rehabilitation, mine after a hip replacement and Neena's after a knee replacement. Their swimming facility is fantastic and their arts and crafts studios well-equipped, but the rest of the place is furnished like an old peoples' home. More recently, I looked into The Mather, which is being built in a perfect location at the edge of downtown Evanston right near parkland on the shore of Lake Michigan and near Northwestern too. I've attended numerous meetings The Mather has held, giving information and publicizing the place. Now the first of the two buildings has been completed and is open to view. So I made an appointment to go on a personal tour today.

It is gorgeous. A real surprise. I am shown apartments with views of the lake to die for. Too small for me to have a studio though, and the place is ridiculously expensive. In addition to passing a financial test, we would have to pass medical tests as well. Residents have to be able to live independently when they move in. I had begun to look into The Mather long before having cancer. Now they might not let me in. It could be a pleasant life though.

Afterwards, I feel frustrated and discouraged. We don't know whether we should stay in Evanston or move to DC, where both our families are nearby.

I discuss it with Lisa, especially about going to DC if Neena should die. She has wanted me to return to the Washington area ever since I moved away. She says I can move in with her, but where? With her ferrets? I suggest buying a larger house in which we all could live, but she loves her house and says that I can live in the lower level. I say I would not want to live in a basement. She suggests adding on.

It's so difficult to plan on being dependent. I think I should stay here unless Neena dies and then move to DC, but live in what kind of place here? And where in DC? Besides, at the rate I am going, Neena will probably outlive me, even though I am four years younger than she is.

OCTOBER 9

It's cold and rainy. Sue has offered to drive me to the weekly OCWW meetings. Since she is president, she goes every week, but I don't go today because she has a cold, and I don't want to be in a closed car with her. I am still protecting myself.

I work on my novel *Borrowed Lives* because Neena's memoir editor wants to read it. Then I do a whole bunch of cooking that knocks me out. I am exhausted and afraid I am coming down with something. I try to straighten up the house, which is frustrating because Neena doesn't like me to move her stuff. Margherita comes over.

I'm having trouble deciding on the cover for the art therapy book. My editor Isabel has sent me three designs, all of which are good, but none grabs me. I send them out to friends and colleagues all over the place to get other opinions.

OCTOBER 10

Cold again today. Autumn has set in. Tony comes over with flowers. He's a sweet guy. I'd like to become involved in the art therapy studio he and Vicky are planning to establish after graduation, probably next summer. I hope I'll have a life then. I watch a Netflix movie at home that I don't really watch. Neena reaches for my hand from her chair to the sofa where I am trying to read. She is used to my reading and watching TV at the same time, which she cannot understand. I take her hand.

She is smiling at me. "Do you know how much it means to me for us just to be sitting here like this together watching TV?"

I smile back. "Yes, I do." I want us to be able to do this forever.

OCTOBER 11

We go to Costco early to avoid the crowd. It is tiring but I manage. Judith and Claire pick us up for an early Italian dinner at Campagnola, since they've just returned from Italy. They are enthusiastic about The Mather. Neena saw her shrink, and she as well as J & C are convinced Neena should spend her money now, especially since she doesn't need to save it for anyone. Jane Bryant Quinn says that's what your eighties are for too.

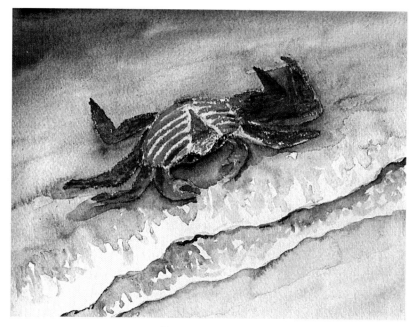

Figures 49. Crab.

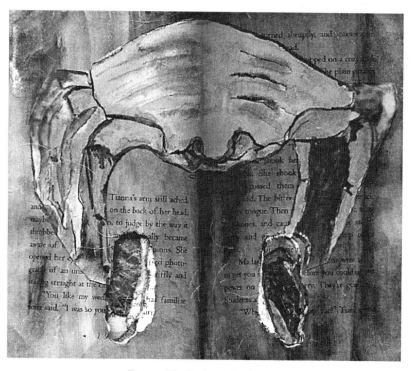

Figure 50. Crab in the book.

OCTOBER 12

I'm jazzed from all the steroids I had to take today. I make granola, clean out and reorganize papers, and calculate expenses, comparing The Mather and present expenses. The Mather is about $30,000/year more, if I don't factor in future nursing home care. I find Illinois expense averages on the Web, and having security about that makes big sense. I try to nap but can't. I work on the altered book. When I'm not feeling so sick, it is easier for me to paint than when I feel horrible. I'm making crab pictures. I look on the Web and discover lots of different kinds of crabs. They are fun to paint. I put one in the altered book.

Neena calls from the annual endocrine minisymposium, where the keynote lecture is named for her, to invite me to join a group of attendees for dinner at the tapas restaurant. I go and eat a ton. The best part is that Laurie, a medical ethicist, is there, across the large round table so I can't talk with her. I do as we are leaving to ask her about the issues in my *Borrowed Lives* novel about a girl conceived to provide a kidney transplant for her brother. Laurie says conceiving a child to donate a kidney for her brother is not a problem, that the second child is often conceived for the first, that she herself was conceived to be a playmate for her brother. Not the same, I think, as surgery for a kidney removal. She wants to read the novel, so I send it to her.

I talk to Gail R. when I get home, the first time in a while. She's all for The Mather. I seem to be poling everyone about what I should do with my life, planning as though I will have one. I like Gail a lot. I'm still jazzed when I go to bed at 10:30 and don't fall asleep until 5:00– 2.5 hours sleep, even with three Ativans.

BLOOD COUNT

Prior to each chemo treatment, my blood gets measured. My doctor needs to know how much has already been destroyed to determine how many more blood cells can be annihilated before I will be killed as well. Red cells contain hemoglobin to carry oxygen. I am tired all the time and I get fatigued from the slightest exertion because my red cells are down, giving me insufficient oxygen. The greatest danger to chemo patients is infection because of compromise to the immune system from diminished white cells. I wash my hands. I use disinfectant wipes whenever I touch anything. I tell friends with colds to stay away. I avoid crowds, i.e., airplanes, movie theaters, plays, and concerts. All those operas, concerts, and plays where I have subscriptions–I've given away the tickets. Chemo kills so much.

At first, I felt strong that although my blood count was low, it was not so low that I couldn't get the full dose of chemo. I didn't want my treatment delayed. My doctor said I was doing fine with it. This was the me I always counted on, just like my brother, knowing I was strong. Now I feel tired and weak, no longer resilient, failing, suffering neuropathy, needing rehydration, demolished.

LAST (I HOPE) CHEMO, OCTOBER 13

Rodriguez says everything looks fine and that I should tell The Mather I am cancer free. He thinks The Mather will let me in. The sore and bleeding on my peritoneum looks like a scratch, he says. How could I get a scratch there? But I'm in the home stretch. I'll have a CAT scan and an appointment with him in three weeks to determine if I am cancer free and then hopefully be done.

"You should live life to the fullest," he says. Maybe he is thinking that I won't have much of it left. "I have a patient who had cancer all through his abdomen so that I couldn't get it all out, but he is still living after seven years," he says. Mine had spread to the omentum and he removed a lot. On the way out, I thank Ann for all she has done for me.

Up in the Kellogg suite, Sally, the psychologist, thinks my Mather plan for a new life is posttraumatic growth. (Maybe it's just denial.) The steroids are revving me up so that I am cheery to everyone. I hope I don't crash, but I probably will in four days as usual. This will be the last time, I hope, I hope, I hope.

OCTOBER 14

I'm feeling pretty good, so I'm taking care of things, picking up a lamp we had rewired with Neena and going to Chaya Sara to fix my wig. The bangs keep getting in my eyes and driving me nuts. I'm being cheery, cheery, cheery.

I take a rest and we go to the opera–*Faust*–my first big theater out-
ing. The chemo hasn't taken effect yet, so I figure I am pretty safe.
Neena loses it in the garage, arguing with the woman in charge, who
tells her to move out of the space she is in. I sweet-talk her. She says
Neena is a "mean one," but I am okay. At dinner, I talk with Neena
about not being able to win a battle with low level people in authori-
ty, like garage employees, that the only thing to do is to appeal to their
mercy and be grateful.

At the opera, I lose an eye-piece to my binoculars. The usher tells
me someone turned it in to her and she threw it away, thinking it was
a bottle cap, but she will look through the trash for it and mail it to me
if she finds it (which she very kindly does several days later). Neena is
impatient with my looking for it and talking to the usher during intermission. We leave before the last act and can't get out of the garage
with its new card system. Neena leans on the horn until an attendant
comes. She screams at him, and I poke her and tell her to shut up because he is trying to help us. Driving out, she tells me never to hit her
again (I didn't) and not to talk to her. I tell her not to say a word to me.
Well, it's obvious how much good the dinner discussion did. Neena
had been so sweet to me on the way down. But she can lose it very
easily.

OCTOBER 15

I go to OCWW with Sue for the first time this fall. Patricia Lear
speaks on illness memoirs and workshops my first fifteen pages of this
journal. Sue, who has studied drama for years, volunteers to read it
aloud and does so with much more emotion than I would be able to
do. The group seems moved. I am very gratified. Later, Sue tells me,
"there was not a dry eye." A few people offer suggestions. As is the
custom, since the pieces are read anonymously, Patricia asks if the
author wants to stand. I do. Although cancer is such personal anguish,
I want others to know what my life is now, especially since the writing
seems meaningful to them. This is a first for me. I'm going public with
what I have been writing. I think about publishing it.

Sue and I go to lunch with others from the group afterwards. I
argue with the restaurant manager over my order because it is adver-

tised as lobster pasta, although there is no lobster in it. She takes something off the price, but I don't eat the pasta. I take it home for dinner, but I don't eat it then either because it is not very good.

After all the responses to the three pictures I had sent out for my art therapy book cover, I decide on a totally different picture. The publisher uses it but doesn't show me the mock-up. It is a painting I made of DNA when I was recovering from surgery. I hope it will work.

Neena is gone for the day and evening–I'm glad. I need time for myself. I get lots of calls from the kids, who are worried about me because I have been out when they've called. I'm very tired and don't feel like talking, but I speak with them briefly. I read a book given to me at chemo about after treatment–a real downer. Lots of lingering effects. Neuropathy can get worse and take a year to improve.

I'm very, very tired. No pooh since before chemo, but I don't feel constipated. There are phone messages from The Mather with more apartments to see, but I am not up to it.

OCTOBER 16

I'm tired and weak, starting to feel bad. No poop since before chemo. Margherita was going to come over, but for the first time, I tell her not to. I'm just too depleted to talk with anyone. Neena is being very kind to me. I think she is worried about how incapacitated I seem. I know she feels helpless sometimes in caring for me. I wish I could make her feel better, which of course is what she feels about me.

Food tastes awful. I don't want to eat, I can't eat. But Neena has invited Richard, the editor of her newly completed autobiography, and his wife for dinner. He has been e-mailing me about my novel in progress, *Borrowed Lives,* and I warned him that the period of their coming to Chicago for a conference would coincide with my post-chemo sick spell, but he is anxious to meet me. I tell Neena to pick them up because I feel too weak to go out, even to ride in the car. I am not strong enough to stand in the kitchen and cook either, to say the least, and she doesn't want to, so we order Chinese.

Richard is different from what I had expected from our e-mail exchanges–a large man. I had visualized him slender, almost aesthetic looking. I start out being hostess, but at the table I cave in. A wave of sickness washes over me. I had eaten hardly anything all day and the Chinese food tastes awful to me. The others can see I am sagging. I force some Chinese, feel faint, and can't see. When I put my head down on the table, Neena is convinced that I am passing out. Richard guides me to the sofa in the living room. His arm feels firm and comforting. I sleep on and off while they visit in the backroom. I can't get up or talk to anyone. They have to take a cab to their hotel because Neena thinks I should not be left alone. She wants to call the doctor and take me to the hospital, but I refuse.

TETHERED, OCTOBER 17, 18

Fortunately, I sleep okay, but I have a sore on my perineum and it burns horribly every time I pee, which is often. I wake up feeling more nauseous and weak than I ever have. It takes me two hours to get dressed and come downstairs. I don't know if I should take a laxative. I don't want to poop and stretch the sore more.

The next day I am the same. Helen and a friend stop by. I can't even talk to them. After they leave, Neena panics. She can't take responsibility, she says, and insists on taking me to the ER.

I am put in a corner room with cartoon circus animals running around the ceiling. Outside are the computers where all the staff congregate, so there is gossip going on full blast. Then some little kid is screaming bloody murder. Another kid, Eric the med student, comes in. Under other circumstances I would have told him my son is also Eric, but I'm not up for chitchat. I feel dizzy, faint, weak, and nauseous. My neuropathy has gotten worse, so I can hardly pick up anything without dropping it. I am being taken care of by a med student who looks eleven. Grant, a nurse, comes in—another kid, this one trying to grow a beard—to inject me for a saline drip. I say I need an IV expert because I don't have any veins, and he says he is one. He actually gets it in. I am wheeled to X-ray, get an EKG [electrocardiogram] and a blood draw, and have to give a urine specimen. The Saturday night crowd begins to arrive, and I can hear the joint jumping.

Eventually Dr. Cooper, the ER attending, comes in. He asks me all about my work. I ask about his. He has been doing ER for twenty-two years. I tell him he doesn't look that old, that everyone there looks thirteen. They are, he says. He is fifty-four, old enough to be their parent. I am old enough to be their grandparent, I say. I've been in the ER for hours. I want to go home. He is going to hospitalize me to run a hydration drip and check on infection, the biggest danger to chemo patients. The X-rays and EKG are good, but my hemoglobin is low, and they suspect a urinary tract infection. They have to culture the specimen to find out.

Neena keeps complaining that she is exhausted and has to go home. I insist that she accompany the gurney to my room so she'll know where I am. She says my clothes are still sweaty. When I ask her to hang them up, she can barely manage it. She tires so easily. I am in bed and need stuff where I can reach it, but she wants to go. For the first time since my diagnosis almost five months ago, I begin to cry. I feel so helpless and abandoned.

In the room next door, I can hear a man retching and moaning. That continues the entire time I am there. God knows what I am catching from him. He sounds as though he is strangling and trying to cough up whatever is blocking his airways. I feel so sorry for him.

Yvette, the night nurse, checks me in. She's a large woman with coffee colored skin and a soft Caribbean voice. She calls me Miss Harriet, which is nice. I sleep but get up multiple times to drag my IV pole to the bathroom.

I ask for towels. I'm sure I'll wet the bed during the night because the nursing assistant won't come fast enough to lower the sides of the bed and get me and my pole to the bathroom. I don't. Finally after five days of no movement, I begin to poop every time I pee, all night long.

The next day, I learn to recognize the staff hierarchy by their colors. Nurses wear royal blue. Nursing assistants wear light green and speak some other language. Cleaners wear dark green and don't speak at all. Food service folks wear black vests and introduce themselves as my host. Doctors wear whatever they want. Dr. Varma has on jeans and a T-shirt under his open lab coat and wears a week's growth of beard. Only the lab coat saves him from looking like a hood.

My day nurse is a small dark woman with a crooked mouth and missing teeth. Her voice is like the caw of a crow and I can't understand most of what she says. My IV keeps beeping, which means it isn't working. Grant had put the needle in the crook of my right arm

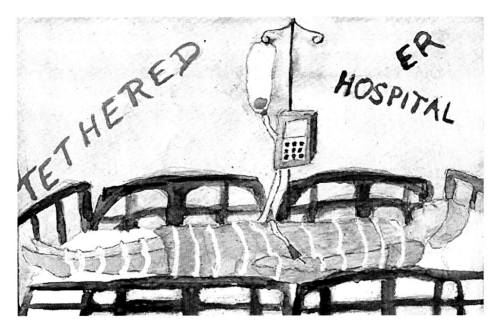

Figure 51. Tethered.

so every time I move it, the tube gets squeezed and the machine beeps. And guess who comes in to fix it–the IV specialist who couldn't get the needle in for my chemo. She does it quickly, but the thing keeps beeping. It is leaking, and once again she didn't get it in. I keep calling my nurse, but she is busy with a patient emergency so I am dripless for hours.

I get hot and cold, sweaty and freezing. I feel weak, sometimes faint, and nauseous. All food tastes awful. My neuropathy is worse, my fingers and toes numb stubs. There's no feeling so I drop everything, and I can't turn pages or hold small pills. There's constant feeling in my feet like when a limb goes to sleep and begins to wake. Sometimes there's pain. My bottom is full of sores, some that burn when I pee and some that itch and tickle all night so that I cannot sleep, and I am constipated.

The doc keeps me for another night because the urine culture hasn't finished growing. They are giving me an antibiotic for a suspected urinary infection. Constipation has turned to diarrhea. My hemoglobin is way down, so the attending, Dr. Varma, is considering a blood transfusion. I am stuffing food in an effort to build red blood cells so I won't have to get the transfusion. Who knows what I'll pick up from the blood? My red cell level goes up a little then down again, but since I am feeling better, he decides not to do it. I am a pin cushion, being stuck all the time with anti-blood coagulant, neuprin to boost my white blood cells, and frequent blood drawings.

I have diarrhea at night and the bed sides are up, so I can't get out. I call for help, but no one comes. I climb out over the railing, IV pole and all. When the nursing assistant finally comes into the bathroom, she says I shouldn't have done that.

"You wouldn't have been too happy if I had pooped all over the bed," I counter.

OCTOBER 19

After two days of being tethered to the hydration IV, I am discharged. I don't have a urinary infection after all. Sonny calls about my coming to Florida next week where he and Joan have rented a condo, but I tell him I just got out of the hospital and won't be able even to think about travel until I feel better. He speaks again of a new chemo for kidney cancer with few side effects that he will take if he needs it again. I don't see how I would be able to go through chemo again, and I am eaten up with anxiety about the upcoming CAT scan to determine if the treatment has worked, in other words, if I am cancer free. Can I have a life again?

OCTOBER 20

I can't sleep because my bottom hurts or itches all night. I have to go to Kellogg for a shot to boost my white blood cells.

In the evening, I attend the Northwestern Emeritus dinner with Neena. I am particularly eager to go because Dominick Messini, a big gun in the Northwestern theatre department, will be speaking about Leonard Bernstein's *The Mass,* which he will direct as his last production before retirement. I had heard that he has cancer. I speak up about seeing *The Mass* when it opened the Kennedy Center, which interests Dominick. I'm very eager to see his production.

Winnie greets me, saying she thought I would lose my hair, but that it looks beautiful. I simply say thank you because, after all, it is my hair, even if in wig form. She says she will never be off chemo. I'm glad she's well enough to attend the dinner though.

I've been reading Katherine Rich's *The Red Devil* (2000), and in it her doctor is telling her about a bone marrow transplant, new in 1989. I'm resisting reading on, too scary.

OCTOBER 21–24

Faygie comes over with mushroom soup–delicious–and her guitar. She sings a butterfly song. I read over The Mather agreement–big problems. Maybe it won't work.

I have an appointment with my internist, Valli Stewart. She takes me off blood pressure medication because I have lost weight, about thirty-five pounds. I hope I can keep it off, but I've been trying to stuff

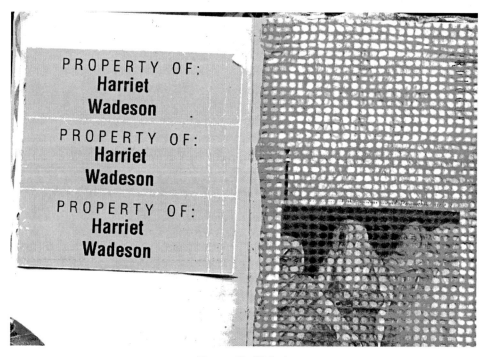

Figure 52. Veiled.

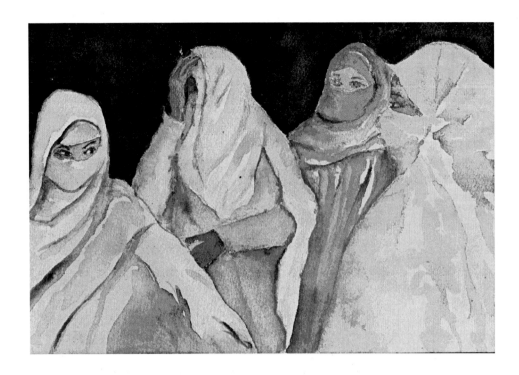

Figure 53. Muslim women.

food to build blood. It is good to see Stewart. She answers lots of questions.

This afternoon I work on a painting for the altered book to relax and enjoy myself. It's an image of Muslim women, veiled and oppressed. My uterine cancer is a women's disease. I reduce the painting on the computer, print it out, and glue it onto one of the introductory pages. Then I cover it with a veil. Until recently, "female problems" were veiled.

It's paradoxical that painting is such a pleasurable experience for me that I feel good even when creating what feels the worst, such as "Chemo Stomach," "Chemo Brain," and "Neuropathy." The latter two were particularly satisfying to make. "Chemo Brain" is a very simple collage, but I like its surreal nature and I think it conveys my experience. For "Neuropathy," I like cutting up other paintings to use in a different way and adding the photograph of a mask I'd made to express the emotion. The same is true for my picture of "Chemo." (*See* Figures 22, 28, and 34.)

I am still depressed. I'll be less so if and when I feel better physically. I am so destroyed by the chemo. It's cold and rainy and my white blood cell count is down. I don't want to risk catching something in a crowd so I have given away my ticket to the opening play at the Goodman Theatre, and Neena has gone with Judith and Claire, who have the series with us.

I go to the Farmers Market with Fran and Bill. I can't go by myself. It looks empty like the cold rainy day. Margherita comes over and we go to Schaefer's Wine Shop for their Saturday tasting, which is also sort of meager. She visits and wants to see my altered book again. I'm glad she finds it interesting. She has become a good friend.

After all the rain, we have a gorgeous sunny day, so Neena and I go to the Botanic Gardens and visit the new science building, because it is the last day for the free shuttle from the entrance and too far for me to walk. It's a nice building with interesting interactive exhibits. But I get tired and feel weak. I have to eat, so I grab some soup in the cafeteria. I don't have the energy to look over the other food. We walk around some, but mostly I sit. There are spectacular autumn blaze pear trees with leaves of vivid purple, orange, and gold, all on each tree. I'm too tired to stay for Halloween festivities, which I would love ordinarily.

OCTOBER 25, 26

I spend four hours looking at Mather apartments. I feel "on," talking nonstop to Mary, the sales representative. Neena comes after two hours. Some of the views are spectacular, over the lake and city in the distance. I pick out the apartment I want, on the top floor with tall arched windows overlooking the lake. Like the others, it is a two-bedroom, too small for me to have a studio. I insist of seeing the nursing care unit, which others probably overlook in their excitement over the gorgeous lobby, library, and dining rooms. It is pretty dismal, without closets in the bedrooms. Those at death's doorstep aren't expected to have possessions. The journey they're on doesn't allow carry ons.

After we are treated to an elegant lunch in one of the seven beautiful dining rooms, Neena takes me aside to tell me that my wig has slid to the side of my head. I wonder if Mary has noticed. She is explaining again that in addition to passing a financial test, prospective residents must pass a medical test to prove they are capable of independent living. My cancer might make me unacceptable, and with my wig askew, Mary might flunk me without even seeing my medical report.

I am exhausted in the evening and feeling awful. I have a nosebleed and sore gums.

The next morning, I wake up obsessing about how to arrange The Mather apartment space, which is too small. I am living in two worlds, one in which the cancer has been treated and I will have a life, and the other in which the only life I will have will be that of a cancer patient. As I wrestle with decisions, Lisa calls and provides the best advice. She reminds me that I need this time to heal, not to move. So true.

Neena and I discuss The Mather. I can tell she expects a battle. She says she couldn't sleep for thinking about it. She doesn't want to move and says we can buy services rather than spending all that money on The Mather. I agree. I think she is greatly relieved. I tell her I want to unclutter this house. I will clear out the shelves in the dining room so she can put her recorder stuff there rather than leaving all her music paraphernalia on the table and settee. I had suggested that she turn the extra room upstairs into her music room, but she doesn't want to. I've started throwing away junk. If I can do a couple of bags every day, maybe I can clear a lot out.

I feel as though my life is on hold until I get the CAT scan results next week. I am so anxious, it is hard to think of anything else. I come back to Lisa's point that I need to use this year to heal from chemo rather than have the stress of moving. I suppose looking at the Mather is an attempt to give my life the continuity it had before my cancer diagnosis. It's like "life as usual," as though having cancer is just an interruption, not a life sentence. I wonder if this flurry over The Mather is just denial and that I won't even have that much life left for a life-care center.

Neena hasn't wanted me to drive, so she insists on watching me drive, i.e., pass a test driving the few blocks to the drug store.

The nosebleed and sore gums are gone, but my neuropathy is much worse. There are so many things I can't do with my hands anymore.

OCTOBER 28–30

Chaya Sara cuts the bangs on my wig and I wear it to Portia. For the first time it feels comfortable on my head and does not slide around, because Chaya Sara has sewn elastic into it.

The Portia folks like it and say I look like Mary Travis of Peter, Paul, and Mary. I wonder if they mean the old Mary or the young one. The older Mary looks like an old hippie to me. I say I am trying to become Ellen (who has long blond hair and also looks like a hippie). She laughs. Cynthia presents details about her conservation work on an El Greco at the Art Institute of Chicago. I am amazed that she is not too intimidated to touch up an actual El Greco. I am fascinated by all her research for work on the painting, but I am so fatigued that I doze and wake to people taking the water glass from my hand.

More decluttering–bags of papers, all health materials. Helen takes Neena and me out to lunch at Ruby's Thai restaurant. The food is too spicy for me. It's pouring rain. Afterwards, I am exhausted and fall asleep at my computer then nap in the backroom. I'm anxious about the CAT scan in a couple days. My life is on hold. People want me to make plans for next week, but I can't until I know the results. Will I have a life? I feel optimistic, but I can't even plan for Eric's visit at Thanksgiving until I know. I finish reading *The Red Devil* (Rich, 2000). It's such a scary book. The cancer spread to Rich's bones and she had a bone marrow transplant and many chemos, but she lived to tell the story ten years later, despite many recurrences. The book didn't seem to have any real ending though. Maybe that's because cancer doesn't, except death.

OCTOBER 31

Happy Halloween. Boo! Robinlee was supposed to come over to work on our AATA conference presentation, but her partner Tracey hacked off the end of her finger. Yuk!

I organize all my cancer papers in files and put them in a file drawer I had cleaned out. I am hoping to be done with them.

People want to get together–Mary Jo, Margherita, Gail R., Goldie, Judith and Claire–but I am waiting to see how I feel after I get the

CAT scan results. The Portia group wants me to let them know the results, but how can I if they're bad? Of course, the kids want to know.

I go to Schaefer's for their Saturday wine and food tasting and walk around the block, then feed trick-or-treaters. From our house, we watch fireworks at the Northwestern stadium in the next block.

The day after tomorrow. . . .

NOVEMBER 1

Robinlee comes over for us to work on our AATA presentation. We write a song, but don't get much more done. She doesn't like my wig. It doesn't look like me, she says.

I am tanking up on water and tea to protect my kidneys from the dye I have to drink for my CAT scan tomorrow. My internist is worried about my kidneys handling the dye. Peeing a lot. Nevertheless, I manage to write a short ditty:

I have joined my father and my brother,
But not my mother.
Like the boys, I now am bald.

I am hot-headed, I am told,
But now my head is always cold.
I feel as though my life has stalled.

Despite wigs and many a hat,
You can be quite certain that
I never get mistook.

Without an eyelash or eyebrow,
Like a cue ball now,
I have that pathetic cancer look.

CAT SCAN, NOVEMBER 2

I was up a lot last night: CAT scan anxiety and having to pee. I drank smoothie dye last night and something bitter mixed with water this morning. They take me right away, so the whole thing doesn't last

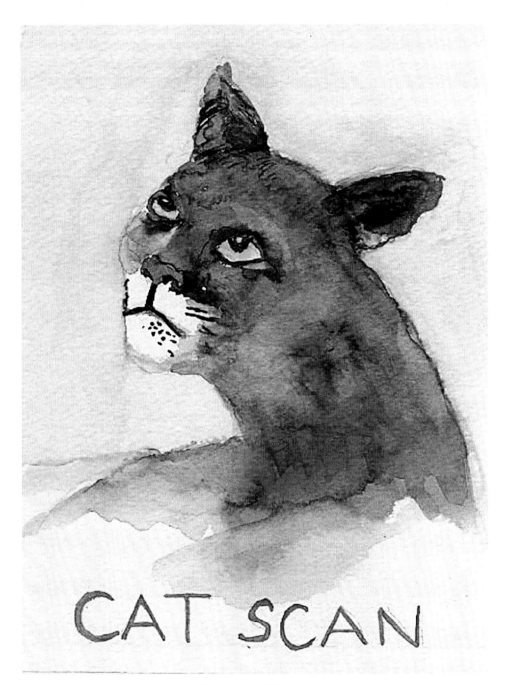

Figure 54. CAT scan.

very long. First, I have to have an IV with more dye. The stuff I drank lights up my colon. The IV is for everything else. I feel it course through me like a heat wave. I lie on a table that slides in and out of the X-ray machine. A smiley face lights up and a voice tells me to stop breathing. I know the routine from before my surgery.

I don't know what to do when I get home. Our yard man removes the large plants in the dining room. I work on the altered book this afternoon. I paint myself tethered to the infusion pole in the hospital. I want to finish the book, but I have to wait for the CAT scan results so I can include a picture of whether I end all this treatment cancer free or not. I want to finish this journal too and the book that may come from it. Mostly I want to end treatment and have a life. It's a sunny day, so for the first time I walk through the golf course to the bridge over the canal, my usual walk before cancer.

Ann said she'd call me this afternoon with the scan results. As the afternoon darkens into evening I get more and more anxious. She doesn't call. I figure: she forgot, she was too busy, the results weren't ready, or the news was bad and she didn't want to inform me over the phone. I tell Neena my concern, and she says that she is anxious too.

When I was teaching at the University of Houston thirty years ago, the Sunday *Houston Chronicle* ran a column by a woman who had cancer, giving advice about how to respond with sensitivity to a cancer patient. In her picture, she looked like a relatively young woman, about my age then. She explained what patients needed and what life was like for them. There was nothing maudlin or angry in what she had to say. One day when I picked up the paper and flipped the pages to her column, she was saying goodbye. "My time has come," she wrote. I felt as though I was losing a friend.

I don't know why I was drawn to reading her back then. Perhaps it was her simple honesty, or more likely, her positive action in the face of her adversity. I think of her now and feel for her all over again, these many years later. Will I one day write, "My time has come?"

MOMENT OF TRUTH, NOVEMBER 3

I actually slept last night. Walking in to the examining room, I pass a small room where I see Rodriguez from the back. He is leaning into a computer, studying a scan. It is a moment's glimpse, but his position appears tense. Is he studying my results? Ann apologizes for not calling me yesterday. The results were not available when she left, and yes, Dr. Rodriguez is getting them now.

He comes in and introduces yet another resident and starts to make chitchat, but I cut to the chase: "What are my CAT scan results?" I expect them to be one way or another, either showing a tumor or clear, but of course they are neither. There are a few suspicious areas that he thinks are probably nothing, a thickening near my umbilicus (probably from previous hernia surgery, I think), a spot on my liver that may have been too small to show up in the previous scan, and an enlarged lymph node in my right pelvis. He says he had taken out many lymph nodes that were clear—thirty-seven, I remind him—so this one is probably a cyst. There is a choice of three ways to find out:

1. A biopsy that would be hard to get because my hip replacement blocks the area
2. A PET scan that can show false-positives because it picks up inflammation
3. Wait three months for another CAT scan to see if it has grown. He seems to lean toward this one, but says it is my decision, not a medical decision, but a personal one. I ask what he would recommend if it was his mother. He says he loves his mother, but it would be her decision.

I ask what the treatment would be if there is more cancer. He says not surgery, chemo—Doxil once a month for six months. I ask about side effects. Sores on the palms and soles, but no nausea. At home I look Doxil up on Wikipedia. It lists nausea and vomiting, hand and foot sores, hair loss, and sometimes cardiac impairment leading to heart failure. It's called The Red Devil or Red Death because the hands turn red. This is the poison Katherine Rich, the author of *The Red Devil* (2000), was taking. She was vomiting a lot. When she had my drug, Taxol, she found it milder! All this makes me wonder how much I can trust Rodriguez. It would make sense that the treatment would get harsher and harsher. I might refuse it.

I e-mail Stewart, my internist, twice, asking about a PET scan. She replies that it's not as bad as a CAT scan on the kidneys and tells me what I already know about false positives from inflammation.

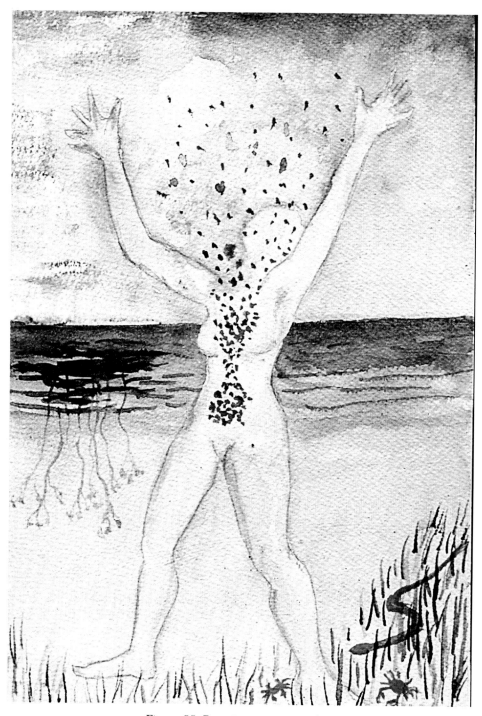

Figure 55. Reaction to scan results.

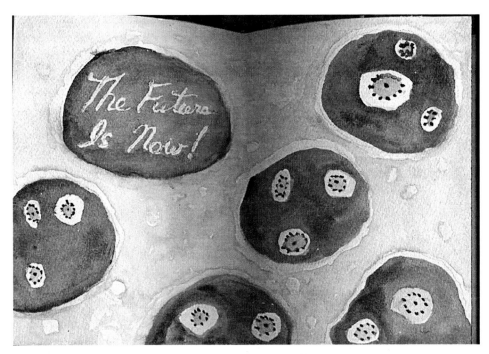

Figure 56. The Future is Now.

So maybe I have something and maybe I don't. No release from anxiety and dread here.

NOVEMBER 4–7

I am doing more as I have more energy. I drive myself to a tai chi class. It is repetitive and boring, not like the tai chi with forms I do in Door County and have done elsewhere.

I go to the Cancer Wellness Center to see Barbara, a personal trainer. I like her. She says I am stronger than I think and that I am doing wonderfully. She has me slide down the big ball with my back arched, which I didn't expect to be able to do.

I have a massage at Evanston Hospital that is good. On the way out, I discover Claire S. in the waiting area of outpatient surgery, where her daughter is having a gallbladder removal. We chat for about half an hour until her husband comes.

I go back in the afternoon to meet with a nurse for a cancer follow-

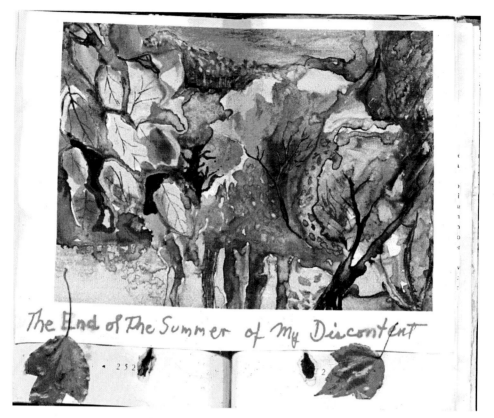

The End of The Summer of My Discontent

Figure 57. End of my summer of discontent.

up program. She tells me things I don't want to hear about developing lymphodemia, swelling of the legs, that radiation can lead to pelvic fracture, that some people don't develop neuropathy until chemo is over, so I guess that means mine could get even worse. In fact it is worse this week and my fingernails are yellowing. I ask about Doxil and she looks it up. An additional side effect is red urine.

So what is this program for anyway? To warn you that you are never free of cancer? That there are always more unimagined torments that can be visited upon you? Why frighten patients with horrid possibilities instead of just dealing with them if they arise and otherwise not scaring those of us who have already lived through terror?

When I ask the survivor nurse about a PET scan, she says my body probably has lots of inflammation now from surgery, chemo, and radiation.

I also ask Sonny about PET scans. He had one years ago with ambiguous results. Joan says that when you have cancer you never get a clean slate, that there is always danger of recurrence, so you should just forget about it during the three months between scans and have a positive attitude. I guess that is what Sonny does, but he is having sciatic pain now and trouble breathing because of his allergies. Joan says his hearing has gotten so bad he couldn't understand a play last night. I wonder if that is due to the chemo or radiation he's had. Neena says my hearing has gotten worse.

Neena has made an appointment for cataract surgery at the end of January. She has been putting it off while taking care of me. I'll be due for another CAT scan right afterwards. God knows what will happen if I am not okay and she has just had surgery.

Robinlee comes over and we work on our AATA presentation. I guess I am going to Dallas in a few weeks. I glue a picture into my altered book that to me looks like autumn exuberance to signal "The End of my Summer of Discontent."

MENDOZA, NOVEMBER 11

I see the integrative medicine doctor, Leslie Mendoza-Temple. I like her. She is very sweet, as well as being beautiful. She encourages recovery, rather than the PET scan, and suggests using this time to be healthy and happy and to make myself strong if I do need more treatment. That makes sense to me.

I have a dream of ordering peanut chews like I ate as a child in the Saturday afternoon movies. In the dream my cancer has spread so nothing matters anymore, and I eat whatever I want. A dream of regression at a time like this makes sense to me.

I slip into the decision of doing nothing but wait until the next CAT scan. Avoidance feels better than pursuit. I hope it's not a fatal decision. I make lots of appointments, for acupuncture, physical therapy, personal trainer, etc.

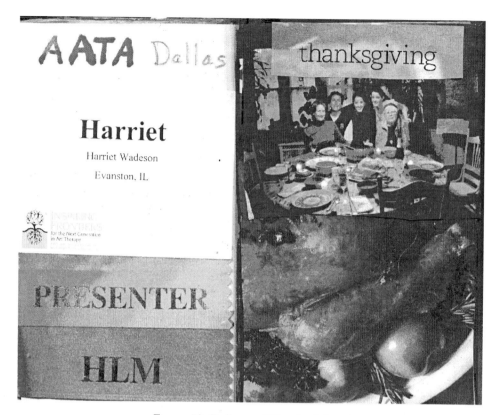

Figure 58. Dallas and Thanksgiving.

DECEMBER 1

I have stopped trying to journal every day. I feel recovered. I went to the AATA conference in Dallas. Neena insisted that I was not to travel alone, so Tony and Vicky looked after me. Nevertheless, I had no problems traveling or attending meetings. It was wonderful to be greeted very warmly by many old friends who told me how glad they were I was able to come. Robinlee and I gave our presentation successfully. My only problem was having to wear my wig the entire time. I shared a room with Gail R., which was a nice opportunity to be with her. We don't see each other often because I live north of the city and she lives way south. I wore a hat to bed as usual, so she never saw my denuded bald head.

I had had enough conference and decided to leave early to attend Helen's eighty-ninth birthday party at home. I was able to manage getting ground transportation and changing my flight at the confusing airport without problems, and I was okay flying home without Tony and Vicky. Helen kept telling me how "dear" I was to come home early for her party.

Best of all has been Thanksgiving with Eric and family. I knocked myself out cooking and we did lots more: theater, Botanic Gardens Winter Wonderland, restaurants, and walks at the lighthouse and Northwestern lagoon. Granddaughters Michaela and Amanda and I made art together, and I helped Michaela get her homework assignments on the computer. At one point when we were at the Botanic Gardens, she gave me a hug impulsively and knocked my wig off. She felt badly, but I told her to forget it. The girls are just delightful, and I have promised Michaela that I will come to California for her high school graduation in June, even though that is a long way off and I don't know how I will be by then. So I guess such a promise is a leap of hope and faith.

I have almost all my old energy back and I am feeling good. It seems fitting to end this cancer journal with Thanksgiving.

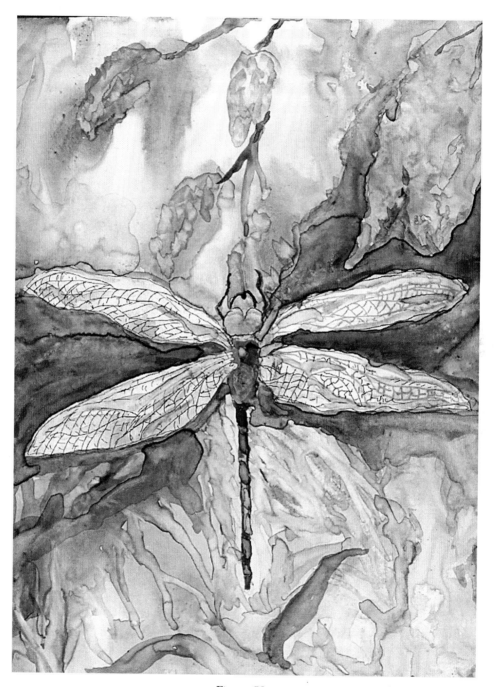

Figure 59.

4

SURVIVING

I realize that the impact of cancer does not end with the completion of treatment or the return to feeling well. There is more, much more. So although I have finished writing the journal on a daily basis, I am continuing to write when I have something to say and the spirit moves me.

DREAD OR DENIAL

I have an overglaze of knowledge about my condition: my cancer is a highly aggressive kind with an 80 percent chance of recurrence in the first years. It is the type of cancer usually found in the ovaries, and it had spread. This understanding is, as I have said, only a glaze. Deep down I believe that it was caught early enough to be eradicated. Deep down, I feel healthy, full of energy, not like a dead woman walking. I am beginning to forget the ravages of chemo and enjoy my full dose of energy, pumped up even more than before I was diagnosed with cancer.

As a therapist, I have been taught to look askance at denial, but it has become my way of life. I am a big fan, the Queen of de-Nile. Otherwise, I would be forced to live in dread. I do not believe there is a healthy middle ground of hope that encompasses a full awareness of the horrendous possibilities.

Dread is life sucking. I recommend denial for all of us who live in Cancer Land. Just so I won't get too carried away, I still have the constant reminders of the pebbles in my shoes from neuropathy and the discoloration and grooves in my fingernails. I watch the changes in my fingernails with a morbid fascination, even as all the health care professionals point to the innocent pink of their lower portions, "See, it's growing out." They sail on de-Nile too.

COUPLES THERAPY

Early in my treatment I suggested to Neena that we avail ourselves of the couple therapy offered by the Cancer Wellness Center to deal with all the stress cancer had been imposing on our relationship. Couple therapy at the Wellness Center is a six-session program with a set topic for each week. I was skeptical, and Neena was worried that because I am a therapist, the couple therapist and I would gang up against her. So we weren't too disappointed when we couldn't be scheduled until after my chemotherapy had ended.

We both feel more positive about it now that it has begun. Megan McMahon, the therapist, tries to help us untangle the knot of our relationship one strand at a time. The first strand is about what has changed in our relationship since the cancer diagnosis. I note that Neena is showing more care, concern, and consideration and that as I result, I have become more appreciative of her. I felt more helpless in relationship to her after surgery and during chemo. Neena says that she has become more considerate of my differences from her and that I have become less patient with her (true).

The second strand is communication. Neena speaks of how difficult it is for her to express her fear of driving at night due to her cataract, for which she needs surgery, and her sadness about my illness, bringing tears to her eyes. I speak of the difficulty I have in voicing my criticisms and what I want her to change, because she gets defensive and offensive. Megan asks what we want from each other. I say caring, concern, understanding, and love. Neena wants me to be well. I respond with how much I appreciate all she is doing to take care of things, such as shopping, cooking, cleaning up, and driving me to the hospital for my frequent visits.

I've conducted a fair amount of couple therapy, and I know how difficult it can be for the therapist to avoid taking sides. I find Megan, though young, to be very evenhanded. At one point, however, she just isn't connecting, so I tell her I am going to give her a little supervision, which is pretty arrogant of me. On the whole, though, I think she is very good and that the therapy is a positive experience for us. We can probably use a lot more of it, but six sessions are all the Wellness Center offers.

Much later, Neena tells me that the sessions were important to her because they were her only opportunity to talk with anyone about how devastated, anxious, and frightened she felt.

READING CANCER BIOGRAPHIES

During the course of my treatment and afterwards, I wanted to read of others' experiences with cancer, although there were many times when I was feeling so sick from chemo that reading the horrors of others' illnesses amplified my own dread to such an extent that I had to stop. Nevertheless, I always returned to the reading eventually with a hunger to learn more about surviving (or not) in Cancer Land.

When I attended the OCWW presentation by Patricia Lear on memoirs of those affected by serious illness, she recommended as a "classic" *The Red Devil* by Katherine Rich (2000). This poor woman went through so many horrors of cancer treatment that her book was difficult for me to read. Despite cancer recurrences and bone marrow transplants, she lived to tell the story ten years later.

Nine years ago, I taught in Italy with noted author Marilyn French. I believe she was my age, or maybe a year older, but she was not well. She had a heart condition and she had had cancer. I was horrified when she told me that, even after she had warned the masseuse before a massage to be careful because her bones were weakened from cancer treatment, the masseuse broke her back. She wrote *A Season in Hell* (1998) about her cancer experience, so as soon as I returned home, I purchased it. I could not read very far in this slim book; it was too painful. This was when I still felt safe, coming as I do from long-lived, cancer-free parents. Now I have a yearning to read it.

I search my bookcases and boxes of stuff to give away for *A Season in Hell* and find it eventually. Marilyn French suffered for a number of years due to the chemotherapy and radiation that caused great destruction to her body and left her with recurring illnesses. Much of the book describes the insensitivity of many who treated her and the lov-

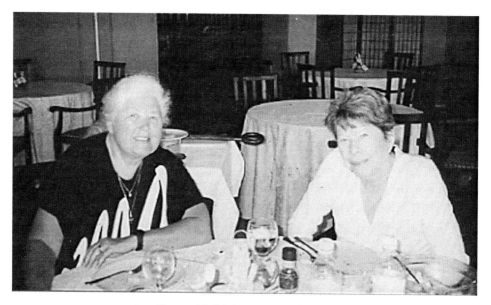

Figure 60. With Marilyn French.

ing care from her children and friends. The book ends with her having arrived at a state of greater serenity where she felt less driven in her life.

Marilyn told me also that she could not write her autobiography until her father, who was ninety-five at the time, had died. She did not expect to outlive him. She died last year at seventy-nine, my age now, and as far as I know, never did publish her autobiography. Her father remains a mystery. I think of my own dilemmas about what to include and what to omit in writing about others. I want it all there. But how can I write some of the things I want to say? Would I be cruel to do so?

I find Lucy Grealy's *Autobiography of a Face* (1994) on Neena's bookshelf and reread it. Her beautiful writing is a pleasure, but the book is more about disfigurement than the other ravages of cancer. In fact, it is doubtful that nine-year-old Lucy even knew that she could die of the disease that robbed her of her lower right jaw. She suffered many unsuccessful reconstructive surgeries throughout her adolescence and wrestled for years with trying to hide what she considered her ugliness.

In *The Cancer Journals* (1980), Audre Lorde's voice as a black woman warrior provides a historical perspective, beginning with her feelings of depression and loss (mastectomy) and evolving to strength and renewed dedication to her work to overcome and eliminate oppression.

Tucked into one of my many bookcases, I find another older memoir I've read: *Cancer in Two Voices* (1991) by Sandra Butler and Barbara Rosenblum, who were partners. It's such a sad book–Barbara died from the breast cancer that was not diagnosed until eighteen months after it showed up on a mammogram, and she had complained to her doctors of symptoms for months. Both she and her partner wrote of their experiences of the cancer. It's a very honest book. Barbara called the money she received from the settlement of her lawsuit against her HMO "blood money." What strikes me now are the two photographs of Barbara. The first is obviously before chemo, in which Barbara's hair is so thick it not only sticks out on the top and sides of her head, but down her face to her glasses as well. Her eyebrows are thick like her hair, and her large glasses cover most of her face. She looks stern. She is wearing a jacket and a heavy turtleneck sweater, so that the overall impression I get is someone very covered up. In the second picture, Barbara is standing in front of Sandy, wearing a lightweight shirt and smiling slightly. Her glasses are perched jauntily on the top of her bald head, and gone are her eyebrows as well as her hair. She looks bare, lighter, somehow stripped down to perhaps her more essential self. Her writing during her last days is like that too. She found a kind of peace after her earlier sorrow and fury, discovering her more essential self, at least as I understand her words.

I pick up the more recent *The Year of Magical Thinking* by Joan Didion (2005), a New York Times bestseller, to reread, although it is not a cancer memoir. Somewhere I read that she completed it in just three months. Her writing is wonderful, and I couldn't put the book down when I first read it. Now after reading a bit, I do put it down. It's about sudden loss and grief and the strange way the mind works in adjusting to the drastic changes they bring about. It's not about my situation, however. Let those close to me read it.

More recent cancer memoirs I've read include *Between Me and the River* by Carrie Host (2009) and *It's Not about the Hair* by Debra Jarvis (2007). Both women went through very difficult ordeals, and Jarvis was a cancer counselor. They are among those with the perfect husbands I mentioned previously.

S. L. Wisenberg, author of *The Adventures of Cancer Bitch* (2009), is a local writer who teaches at Northwestern. I attended a workshop she gave, but I didn't have the *chutzpa* to ask her about either her memoir or her cancer. The book is wry and witty, interspersed with political commentary. Because we teach at the same university and know many of the same people, maybe I'll ask her about it one of these days.

Another recent memoir, though about stroke rather than cancer, is *My Stroke of Insight* by Jill Bolte Taylor (2006), a New York Times bestseller. The author was cared for by her mother during her years of recovery. I had a problem with this author's voice, although I still felt admiration for her and her mother's perseverance during her long slow process of recovery over a number of years.

Currently, I am reading the amazing story of the HeLa cells of Henrietta Lacks, the first line of human cells ever to achieve immortality by continuing to grow outside the body, in *The Immortal Life of Henrietta Lacks* (Skloot, 2010), another *New York Times* bestseller. Scientists had been trying for years to obtain live human cells for experimentation. The cells taken from the cancerous cervix of Henrietta Lacks a few days before she died from the disease in 1951 were named HeLa and not only paved the way, but have been reproduced into the trillions. The quantity is estimated to be large enough to blanket the earth. Henrietta's noncancerous cells, on the other hand, did not survive in the Petri dish. The HeLa cells have been the basis for developing the polio vaccine, chemotherapy (including the Taxol I was given), studies of longevity, the effects of space travel on human cells, and countless other scientific developments.

One of the studies I found particularly interesting was that of telomeres, a string of DNA at the end of each chromosome that shortens every time the cell divides. After approximately fifty divisions, when the telomeres are almost gone, the cells stop dividing and die. The HeLa cells were used to discover an enzyme called telomerase in human cancer cells that rebuilds the telomeres so that the cells can keep regenerating their telomeres and thereby live indefinitely. This seems like a strange paradox to me–that by achieving longevity, thwarting death to become immortal even, cancer cells kill the body.

The book raises significant questions of race (Henrietta was black), class (her family was poor), and medical ethics (the Lacks family was never informed of the multimillion dollar industry developed from

Henrietta's cells). In Skloot's account, they come very much alive.

What has personal relevance for me is a detail I read last night. A review of Henrietta's medical records many years after her death revealed that the nature of her cervical cancer was glandular, not epithelial as diagnosed. She actually had a much more aggressive cancer than originally suspected. The account of her autopsy, describing in visual detail the extensive spread of cancer throughout her body, appears in several parts of the book. I find it terrifying, because the first evidence of my cancer was the appearance of glandular cells, like Henrietta's, in my Pap test, with more glandular cells showing up in the D&C.

Testimony to the reading public's interest in fatal diseases is the extensive history of cancer, *The Emperor of All Maladies* by Siddhartha Mukherjee (2010), another *New York Times* bestseller. I am about 200 pages into the book, shuddering at the barbaric cancer treatments of the past. I have been reading about the radical mastectomies of previous decades that eviscerated women, even removing parts of their necks. Perhaps readers in the future will be horrified to read of the destruction to the body by present-day chemotherapy.

I haven't intended to write a comprehensive review of cancer memoirs and illness accounts here, just the related books that I happened to read or reread during and after my treatment. The one piece of information that would be most specific and informative for me to read, I avoid. It would be so easy to look up my diagnosis, serous papillary carcinoma, on the Internet, but I am afraid. It may be a message of doom and torture, a death sentence.

WORKSHOPS

I am writing this during a cancer journal workshop at a hospital in the city. At least it was advertised as a workshop, but the leader indicates otherwise. So what is it anyway? I never would have driven all the way downtown to spend the evening just to hear the benefits of keeping a journal. Why would any of us be here if we weren't already interested in journaling? Barb, the leader, a fat woman with glasses and frizzy bleached hair, is preaching to the choir. She's a therapist who obviously knows some of the five other participants, probably through her support groups, so she has not introduced herself or asked us to introduce ourselves. I don't know anyone here.

The sales talk on journaling has now gone on for half an hour. I butt in. I interrupt. I ask for what I want. I get us to introduce ourselves. It is hard for Barb to let go of her prepared *spiel.*

She just said, "When do you listen?" Why can't she stop talking and listen? "This is a class, not a workshop," Barb says. In other words, shut up.

Hope springs infernal. After the journal session, I go to another one for women on surviving. I'd read in a cancer manual that once treatment is over, some patients miss their doctors and nurses, but I figure that whoever wrote that we miss our treatment couldn't have had chemo. Who would miss chemo? Right? Wrong! I can hardly believe my ears when one of the women in the session complains that her friends expect her life to be as it was before and that no one brings casseroles anymore. My friends are not like that. They ask how I am. They call after doctor appointments to find out the results. They even bring soup or a cake on occasion. They know I live in treacherous terrain.

To me, these workshops feel like an alien universe where people miss the casserole patrol. It's a place where the women are looking for ways to fill their time, or so they say. I don't seem to have enough time

Lately I have been searching and not finding groups for my own expression, tai chi, art, writing. They're all wrong. Am I so different from others? Where can I find the people I want? I have said that it is kindness that matters, not intelligence or creativity, but now I wonder. My friend Ellen says that therapists need intelligence. I agree.

THREE-MONTH CHECKUP, FEBRUARY

My life is divided into three-month segments, the windows between checkups. I have done nothing to investigate the suspicious spots on my CAT scan of three months ago, following the recommendations of Rodriguez and Mendoza-Temple. My recent CAT scan and Pap test this month, however, show no problems, so with great relief I move out of Cancer Land Center City to an outlying suburb, Limbo Land. I feel great with lots of energy, and I am getting back on track in the activities of my old life. I will be teaching at Northwestern again this spring. Sometimes I can even convince myself that I have moved back into my old life, but most of the time I am aware of the specter that shadows me wherever I go. Limbo Land resembles my old neighborhood, the same houses, the same streets, but the sun is not quite as bright nor the air as fresh.

DEATH, MARCH

In contrast to my own feelings of good health right now is Winnie's decline. I visit Al in a waiting area in Evanston Hospital, where he and Winnie's daughters are holding her death vigil. He looks terrible, wasted and drawn. I don't see Winnie. Her older daughter tells me that Winnie had said she didn't want to linger, but here she is lingering.

A couple of weeks later, Neena and I attend the Quaker-style memorial service for Winnie. She was a lovely woman. Will I follow in her footsteps?

RECOVERY FROM CHEMO, MARCH

I chart my recovery from chemo on my fingernails. They turned hard and yellow with grit the colors of sand and coal dust under them, even though they were not dirty from anything outside my body. Deep grooves have divided each in the middle, bisecting them all in the same place, perhaps the margin between chemo and posttreatment. I have dug at the grit and clipped the ragged ends to remove the crudded part as much as possible. Except for the grooves, which are now two thirds up the nails, they are now almost clear, with only a few showing the jagged margin between the pink part and the white ends. My fingernails have bothered me more than lost hair, even though they are mostly unnoticeable. I see them. From moment to moment, they remind me of the devastation my body has endured from treatment. Their return to almost normal is another small triumph. My body can mend itself.

Of course hair is further evidence. Tonight, I "come out" at the Portia meeting, baring my head without wig or hat. Joanna says I look fabulous and others are equally complimentary. I look as though I am wearing a small white cap with a fringe of curls in the back, much more "with it" than my long mane. My new hair feels like moss, and my head is mossy inside too.

I take the train downtown (which last summer I thought I would never be able to do again) to give an invited speech to the art therapy students at the Art Institute of Chicago and visit the Hollis Sigler Breast Cancer Journal (1999) exhibit at the Cultural Center. Her work is luminous, but the imagery of feminine clothing and objects, such as dressing tables, doesn't do much for me. A woman approaches me to tell me how "snappy" I look in my blue plaid wool beaked cap. It is the one I bought for Daddy in Scotland to match his bright blue eyes. He wore it endlessly until he was no longer here to wear anything. This is the first time I have ever worn it in the fifteen years since his death. It fits me well and is very comfortable, and yes, snappy.

WEIGHT, APRIL 1

I've gained back fifteen of the thirty-five pounds I'd lost. Being thinner was great. I fulfilled my time travel fantasy of going back to younger years when I could fit my bod into the beautiful duds that were gathering dust in my closet, feeling foolish for believing I would ever squeeze into them again. Now I have. More recently, some have become tight again.

Clothes are not the best of it. Walking is. Distances without having to stop and rest. I'm in Door County for the first time since last summer, and today I walk the mossy rocked Lynd Trail along Lake Michigan. I love to sit on those level limestone outcroppings, made soft by moss, and gaze at the water rushing in with great spumes when it is windy and licking the beach peacefully when it is calm. Today, the water howls in relentless waves, and the wind tears through my coat, so I have no wish to sit and gaze. I move on at a fast clip, stepping over rocks and roots without my previous perusal of good sitting places. I don't need them. I can walk without tiring. My clothes are no fantasy. I have re-entered my younger self.

My hair is now a silky white cap. I love it. Everyone else does too. If I take off those fifteen pounds I have gained back, I will be satisfied with my appearance (an unusual condition for a woman in our society), but eating, enjoying my food, savoring it once again, is part of the gusto of returning to life. It is difficult to hold myself back.

PLAYING THE CANCER CARD

The cancer card should not be played at every deal of the hand. I play it, however, for a several thousand dollar tax penalty waiver. I had not paid taxes on government bonds that had matured because I had not redeemed them. So the IRS got me for underpayment of taxes. I appeal the penalty, explaining that because I was undergoing cancer treatment, complete with side effects, I had not understood that taxes were due on the unredeemed bonds, which is true. I enclose a check for the tax due plus interest and request a waiver of the penalty. I get the waiver. The cancer card is a trump.

I also contest a parking ticket I got for failure to display an up-to-date neighborhood parking sticker required for the morning rush hour. Once again, I play the cancer card for failure to notice my sticker is out of date. My appeal is rejected on the basis that I'd had enough time (six months) to replace the old sticker. I truly hadn't noticed, and the only reason I hadn't gotten a ticket before was because I have been parking in the garage because of the demolishment of my previous car by the drunk driver who careened into it when it was parked in front of the house. The ticket is only $30, so I don't appeal the decision.

Sometimes I try to play the cancer card as an excuse for my short temper. It doesn't work. I guess I really don't think cancer is an excuse for anything except feeling bad, but I suppose I still wear the cancer card as sort of a Purple Heart. Wounded in action, but not in the service of my country. I guess I have to say in the service of life.

SIX-MONTH CHECKUP, MAY

Yesterday Ann called to tell me my CA 125, a cancer marker in the blood, is 4.8–way low. Below 30 is good. I am ecstatic. Today I see Rodriguez in the new Evanston Hospital Kellogg Cancer Center wing that was being built the whole time I was in treatment. The new wing is much nicer than the old department. It has a spacious waiting room and a parking lot right outside the door, so there isn't the long twisted walk through hospital corridors with gurneys of very sick people. I want the old department to remain the place of my treatment and the nice new wing to be only a place of checkups for me.

Rodriguez's office and examining rooms are just upstairs. He examines me and finds nothing. I tell him I feel great. "Everyday without chemo is a good day," he says. He is very happy for me, he adds. He's a sweet guy. I have another three-month window of life. As I've said, this is how my life is parceled out, in three-month segments between checkups. I feel good. I feel alive. I am so grateful. I imagine myself years from now thinking this cancer was a wake-up call, a reminder that life is finite, a nudge to make me love the life I have. This is the first time since my diagnosis that I have allowed myself to imagine living long.

Some things never change. Almost a year after my cancer diagnosis, Rachel is still commenting, "I so admire the way you have handled your cancer. You have just been so courageous throughout it all. And you know, people would question your even submitting yourself to all that treatment because you are so old." Right, Rachel, why would old people, who should be dead by this time anyway, want to live!

DC, MAY

After a trial run trip to Florida in January, I am ready to make travel plans once again, but not for the distant future, just for the next few months. My first priority is to see my kids. I had already told granddaughter Michaela I would come to her June graduation in California, so I book DC for spring, azalea time, to see Lisa and Keith.

Lisa loves my hair. She says I am like a little lamb. Keith looks like a hippie. For the first time in his adult life he has let his hair grow out, so now it looks exactly like Lisa's, all puffy with strands of gray among the brown.

In order to look into what moving to Washington might be like for us, I ask Lisa to take Neena and me to visit some retirement communities with my old DC friend Nancy, who is interested also. In one after another, walking question marks push their walkers with effort. We visit the apartment of one lady who complains how far she has to walk from her bedroom to answer her front door, as though her ornately furnished apartment is humongous. All of it could fit into our dining room. Pictures framed on the end tables remind us that once she was a good-looking woman with a beaming smile and a husband. I ask Neena if she wants to live with all these old people.

Even old friends I visit in Washington are beginning to look feeble. Nancy and Rita are still attractive women, but Sonia is wrinkled and wobbly from a hip fracture. She is less sure of herself these days. We get so vulnerable. Roberta, who was always tall, seems smaller. Plastic surgery has given her back her younger face, although drier looking. Her hair that has been so many different colors over the years is thin and colorless. As she grows smaller, her husband Bob gets larger. His red face is more jowls than features. Nancy's husband Mark has now been dead eleven years (cancer), so he probably looks worst of all.

I visit old stomping grounds: the NIH where I worked for thirteen years, Porter Street where I grew up, and Carderock Springs where I lived as an adult. I can hardly find my way around the NIH campus, it is so changed with new buildings and strenuous security prohibitions. The huge Clinical Center, where my office was, is overgrown with add-ons, so that the building I knew is but a central kernel in the now massive edifice. Megan R., the art therapist at NIH, introduces me to her staff as "the goddess of art therapy." It is kind of fun to be a goddess.

I have not been inside the Porter Street house since my parents sold it fifty-five years ago. The owner is wonderfully gracious in letting us come in and look around. The house has shrunk considerably, and the screened porch is now a study, the red brick fireplace is painted white, and the once large kitchen has been modernized with new appliances and granite counters. It looks small, even with the inclusion of the pantry, no longer divided from the kitchen by a wall. I'm pleased to find a few remnants of my childhood, however. The brackets reinforcing the banister are still in place. My father had nailed them to its posts and the floor to stabilize the banister from the weakening Sonny and I caused from sliding down it all the time.

We pull into the driveway of the once beautiful Carderock Springs house but do not go inside. The owners have added on and painted the lovely natural variegated sand-colored brick some ugly shade of pale mud. Time can be told in old houses.

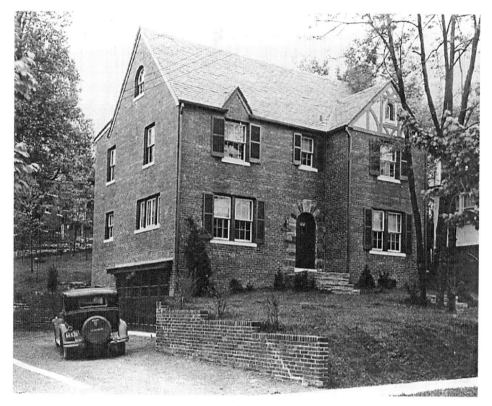

Figure 61. Porter St. in my childhood.

MICHAELA'S GRADUATION, JUNE 10

The California sun is shining on me on this, Michaela's high school graduation day. Her friends and their families are coming and going on the large deck of Eric's house as we toast everyone. Last Thanksgiving when Eric's family visited, I told Michaela I would come to her graduation, wondering if I would be well enough to do so. Here I am, no longer zapped from chemo, feeling good, enjoying life. Michaela is exuberant; it is a delight to see her so happy.

Eric shows me all the pictures stored on his blackberry, including some from Thanksgiving. Those of me in the wig are awful. Although it was made from my own hair, I never looked like myself in it because the hair had been straightened. Hanging in my face or pushed aside, the bangs were ridiculous.

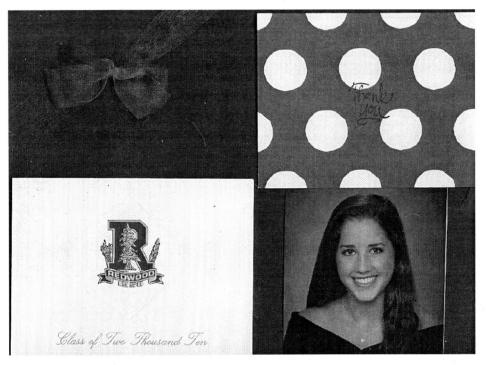

Figure 62. Michaela's graduation.

I add the invitation to Michaela's graduation with the picture she enclosed and her thank you note for my gift to the last page of the altered book. In a way, this is a graduation for me too. A year ago, Rodriguez said that if I didn't have treatment I would be dead in a year, and here I am, a year later, very much alive.

CAREGIVING AND CHILDREN, REVISITED

A high priority for me has been visiting my children now that I can. I know they love me and have felt very concerned about me during this past year. They continue to call me daily, if not more frequently, but I feel increasingly uneasy about my precarious future and worry about whether I will be able to count on them if I should need their help. Neena is elderly and becoming more so each day with health problems of her own. I worry about how we will manage if my cancer should return.

I am so much a product of this society that separates families through the mobility of its members. After all, I am the one who moved away. At the time, I voiced my concern to my parents about them. My father's response was, "Everyone has to grow up and leave home sometime." I was forty-eight. I never thought of myself as the one who would someday need family nearby. As would be the case for my children, it is burden enough to be caring for a declining or gravely ill parent, but to do so from a distance is beyond being a burden, it is a hardship, especially for those who need to work and raise their own children.

Our society is so mixed up around end of life issues. On the one hand, we have developed medical technology to the level where we can lengthen life in even the most hopeless and helpless cases. We have extended longevity so that we have increasing multitudes of elderly individuals needing care. Beyond medical care, we have made few provisions for the emotional and life-care needs of those near the end of their lives. The custodial services for them and the life-care centers that are being built are expensive and therefore out of reach for large segments of our population, who may live in isolation and/or with inadequate care.

We seem not to know what to do with those who are old, ill, or dying. We value life, health, and youth to the extent that we deny the inevitable ends they reach. Certainly, family members responsible for the care of their elders need support and assistance. Those without family who are near the end of their lives need even more.

What is called for is an attitudinal change that can give value to this inevitable phase of life, rather than the dread and denial that are associated with it now. Other cultures have revered their elders and assigned family to care for them. For them, the wisdom and experience of age are respected. Their elderly are not considered obsolete, to be warehoused in some holding environment until they die. In such cultures, families often live together throughout their lives, such as in the family compounds I visited in Bali.

I do not believe I will live long enough to see our societal attitudes towards aging and provisions for the end of life revolutionized. So I need to cast a practical eye on the arrangements Neena and I can make for ourselves now. We are probably among those who are fortunate in being able to afford to pay for help if we should need it. If Neena is no longer here or able to care for me, I do not want to be cared for by a stranger. I want someone who loves me and knows me for what I have been as well as what I am to care for me, perhaps with help from paid assistants. I don't know how to bring that about, short of moving to where one of my children lives. I may have to do that, although it would mean leaving my entire support system. Uprooting is hard for the old; one can't exactly start over in a new place at an advanced age.

I will have to talk with my children about all of this, that much I do know.

POTLUCK, JULY

We are on our way to the potluck with Judith and Claire, this month being held in Michigan. We drive through squalls of rain pummeling the windshield into opacity, punctuated with jagged streaks of lightning and crashes of thunder. Between storms on a dry stretch of the Indiana Skyway, Judith asks me, "Has the cancer changed you? You seem the same in conversation and all."

I don't need even a moment to reflect. "I'm grateful for every day I am alive. There is not a day that goes by that I am not aware of how happy I am to be feeling well. As my doc says, 'A day without chemo is a good day.'"

On the way home, Judith tells us that a mutual friend who arrived at the party just as we were about to leave told her that Claudia is back in chemo, less than a year after she began it before. I feel so badly for her. On the long ride home, I am thinking not only of Claudia. "There but for the grace of God. . . ."

NINE-MONTH CHECKUP, CAT SCAN, JULY 29

I have returned to the circuit. I taught my Northwestern course in the spring, and I conducted a workshop in California in June. All went well. I can still do these things.

It has been six months since my last CAT scan. I am teaching every afternoon at Northwestern this week, so I scheduled the CAT scan and my appointment with Rodriguez to get the results for next week when my class will be finished. I didn't know how I would face my students if I got news that the cancer has recurred. Ann called to say Rodriguez will be going on vacation the day of my appointment, so I rescheduled for two weeks later when he returns, but I have been having stomachaches over the past couple of months and pain in my right breast for the month since my mammogram (which turned out okay). I am filled with fear that they are the result of cancer recurrence and dread that the CAT scan result will be a death sentence. I am eaten alive with anxiety and don't want to wait three weeks to get the verdict. I called and switched the CAT scan to two days ago and the appointment with Rodriguez for today. I'll have to go straight from Rodriguez to the class and just deal with my students and try to be responsible to them even if I am demolished from a verdict of cancer recurrence. It seemed the lesser evil than living longer with this anxiety.

Two nights ago, when we had dinner with Judith and Claire, Judith said that Claudia will never be in remission again, because once ovarian cancer returns it stays. My cancer, serous papillary carcinoma, is the same kind as ovarian cancer. I didn't say this to Judith and Claire. Is this the end of my life, my so very precious life? Will I be able to go to the *Passion Play* in Oberammergau, Germany, next month? That trip I've planned is so special to me, a return to beautiful Bavaria, where I lived in my early twenties.

Two scenarios spin in my head, my relief when Rodriguez will tell me everything is fine, and the death sentence. I remind myself that results are not always clear-cut, maybe something will look suspicious and I will need more tests. I imagine having a life but with punctuations of great anxiety every three months. How will I be able to teach my class at Northwestern right after my appointment if the news is bad? I have moved back into my life. I want to stay here.

Neena and I are sitting in the Kellogg Cancer Center waiting room. I am trying to ready myself for the verdict, a death sentence, a life sentence of patienthood, freedom? As I left the house, I grabbed Norman Cousins' *Anatomy of an Illness* (1970). I had read it years ago and remember his recommending humor and laughter. In the waiting room, I turn to a chapter on creativity and read about Pablo Casals and Albert Schweitzer, who had purpose in life fueled by their creativity. Cousins says that leads to longevity. I visualize Casals and Schweitzer each playing Bach on the piano to uplift myself through their examples. I know creativity leads to feeling better. I think of myself painting my way through cancer and tears swell in my eyes.

I am summoned to the examining room. Ann comes in and hands me pages with columns of figures. "Your numbers are all good," she says, referring to my blood work. "Your CA 125 is way down, which is excellent." This blood test measures a protein released by ovarian cancer cells. I look at my scores. I've passed all the tests. "Dr. Rodriguez is down talking to the radiologist now about your CAT scan results," she adds. Does talking to him instead of just reading the report mean that there is something to talk about? I am partially relieved by the CA 125, but that isn't always an accurate test.

Rodriguez comes in smiling, his usual friendly self.

"I hope you have good news for me," I say.

"Very good. Nothing has changed on your CAT scan since last time." A reprieve, or a stay of execution. Neena and I are both so relieved, and Rodriguez tells me how happy he is for me. He is such a warm, caring doctor. He examines me and finds nothing, not even in my painful breast. He refers me to a breast doctor. "We have tunnel vision," he says. "You need a breast expert. Your stomach pain is in exactly the place of your hernia operation" (near the navel two years ago). He refers me to another doctor for that and tells me I need my regular exam from my internist as well.

As we leave, Neena tells Rodriguez, "You're a good doctor."

I say, "Thank you, you've made my life."

As always, he says, "I'm just the messenger. You should thank God, not me."

In the car, Neena says, "I'm so relieved. I didn't tell you how anxious I was."

"And I didn't see it either. I couldn't have gone through this without you."

When she stops for a red light, she takes my hand. "This is what partners do. How could we possibly live without each other?"

Later in class, I have the worst and longest stomachache yet. I am reminded that just because the cancer has been stopped for now doesn't mean that all other problems have ceased as well. Another cancer legacy: every ache, pain, or twitch is seen as a possible recurrence.

Although I have assigned my students to do an art piece about stressors in their work situations, I draw my cancer crab. It's what I

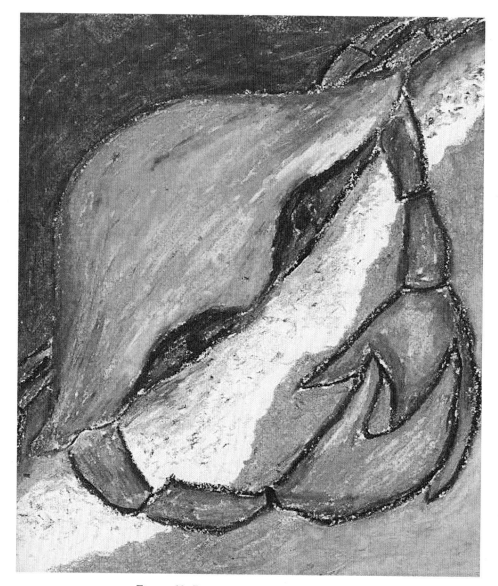

Figure 63. Drawing in Northwestern class.

need to do at that moment. The fear of its return has been such a pervasive stressor. I hadn't planned to talk to the students about my illness, but I have to explain my picture, so I tell them my good news. They are wonderful in expressing their happiness for me.

KARATE, JULY 31

When I was fifty-six, I began training in karate, a little late in the day, you might say. I stuck with it for nine years until I was sixty-five. I progressed slowly, finally attaining the rank of brown belt, one step below black belt. Often, I found myself sparring with 20-year-olds, a somewhat daunting experience. I haven't trained in karate in almost 15 years, but tonight I am attending the dojo's twenty-fifth anniversary party. It has grown in many ways, including size and programs offered, since its early days when I was a white belt.

I drive with trepidation to the pub where the party is being held. I don't expect to know people there and imagine myself just standing around looking on at partyers having a good time with all their buddies. The director ("Sensai") greets me warmly with a hug. Shortly after I began training, she was diagnosed with breast cancer. Right after coming home from the hospital where she'd had a mastectomy, she did four hours nonstop of kata (karate forms, like dances). She looked beautiful bald and never missed a class. She is a wonderful example of recovery. I tell her I am now in her league, having also lost my hair.

People whose names I don't remember and whom I don't expect to remember me rush over to hug me. The party organizer ushers me in front of others and gets me a chair to hear the speeches. I am treated like an honored guest. One youngish woman whom I don't recognize at first tells me how important I was to her in her training. I'm surprised. How? I ask. She explains that it was the way I befriended her. She puts her arm around me and we stand that way for a long time while we watch old slides of us sparring and performing katas.

What am I trying to say here? I had felt so insignificant in the dojo. I was by far the oldest person there throughout those nine years, often feeling obsolete, out of it. Our dojo was so much about physical prowess and fighting spirit. It's such a surprise to me that today many consider me to have been a valued member of the dojo. It is warming that they are genuinely happy to see me. At times like this, my self-knowledge seems very limited.

LIFE GOES ON

Neena and I attend a potluck given by a new organization Neena has joined for people who want to age in their own homes. Al has joined too, and the party is being held in his new apartment. He looks good, and the apartment is spacious and attractive with lots of Native American weavings on the walls and Native objects on the tables and floor. Al tells me that Winnie decorated it and was able to complete it before she died. She got to live in it only a few months, but life goes on and so it will after I have gone as well.

PASSION PLAY, SEPTEMBER

I have a very good three-month segment before my next checkup. Best of all is my Germany adventure. Last winter, my son-in-law Mark and I decided to go to the *Passion Play* in Oberammergau, which is given only every ten years. I figured, now or never. I doubt I'll be able to make it in ten years when I am eighty-nine, if I live that long.

Four hundred or so years ago, the villagers there prayed to be spared from the plague, promising to put on a *Passion Play* every ten years if they were. They have done so ever since, with everyone from the village taking part. We had to purchase tickets months in advance, which was an act of faith for me. I tried to talk Lisa into going, but she hates to fly. So it is just Mark and me. (How many guys want to travel with their mother-in-law?)

Mark is the perfect traveling companion. He carries my suitcase, does the driving, and speaks in German so that he improves upon my halting Deutsch. I enjoy getting to know him a lot better through our lively discussions as we drive from town to town. The *Passion Play* is wonderful, as are the charming alpine villages and the beautiful mountains. Mark does lots of hiking, while I take ski lifts. At one of the lovely mountain lakes, a ferocious swan attacks me, hissing and threatening to bite me. I didn't know I could jump so fast. Swans are such graceful creatures, I never would have expected such viciousness. After Mark leaves, I speak to German art therapists in Munich, where they take me to the Oktoberfest. It is another trip down Memory Lane, because I lived in Munich in my twenties. Do these returns to places of my youth signal end-of-life review?

GOING PUBLIC PROFESSIONALLY, NOVEMBER 4

Shortly before my one year checkup, I go to Sacramento for the AATA Annual Conference in order to present my cancer altered book that is included here. This is my opportunity to see if my cancer artwork can fly professionally. Although I have done too many presentations to get nervous about them anymore, I do have anxiety about this one since the art is mine and it is so personal. I play to a packed house and get a wonderfully positive response, which encourages me to go ahead with publication. Being thanked for the presentation by so many people is immensely gratifying. During the rest of the conference, people approach me to tell me they have had cancer or their mother had and they had never known before what chemo was like for her. The cancer community is large indeed.

RETURNING TO MY LIFE: MY LIFE RETURNING TO ME

I completed my cancer treatment one year ago. In time I have come back. Once again, I am strong. I have energy. My appetite has returned, as has some of my weight, with gusto. My fingernails are no longer grungy, looking dirty, and discolored. They have returned to their pretty pink selves with distinct margins. The peripheral neuropathy remains, however, a perpetual tingling reminder that my body has been assaulted. I've had it over a year now, so the damage is probably permanent. It is an invisible sign. The most prominent visible manifestation of my progress is the bunch of curls sprouting from my head that everyone loves, telling me I look younger. I've even had to trim my hair, snipping soft white tufts from the nape of my neck and around my ears. On the back cover of my altered book, I glue pictures showing the progression of my hair growth. This is the ending of my altered book, which has now become too full to close.

I have survived not only cancer, which I never even noticed, but the chemotherapy that was destroying my body. I live in gratitude for each day, each minute, that I am vital, that I feel well. There is not a moment of feeling healthy that I take for granted. I know these moments are finite, that at any time I may need more chemotherapy to begin destroying me again, but I am trying to live each moment fully, grateful for what is now.

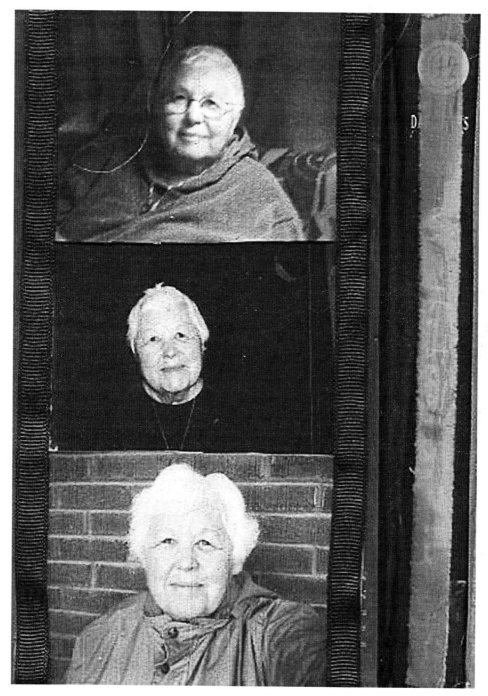

Figure 64. Back cover: Hair growth.

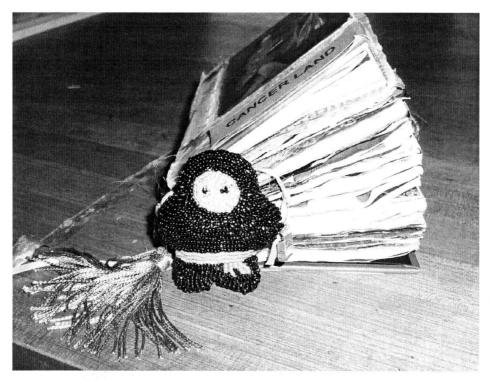

Figure 65. A full book.

This feels like a good place to end this journal, with the addition of my one year checkup to round it off.

ONE YEAR CHECK-UP, NOVEMBER

I arrive at my one-year checkup confident from the low level of my CA 125 report, which I have seen already. Since my last appointment with Rodriguez, I have followed up on my breast and stomach pains. The breast doctor found nothing, but I did. The seat belt in my car was pressing into my breast. That was an easy adjustment. The gut guy said a hernia operation would be discretionary. Since I've had enough insult to my body recently, I am not contemplating more surgery now. So I enter the Kellogg Cancer Center without the apprehension I've had at past checkups.

When Rodriguez comes into the examining room, I am not anxiously awaiting dire test results, so I chat with him briefly. I tell him about my Oberammergau trip and ask him about his life. I am feeling very chipper, but in his internal examination, Rodriguez finds a spot.

"It's probably nothing," he says as he cuts into it for a biopsy. "I'll put some silver nitrate on it. It won't hurt." It stings and burns. He leaves and I get dressed, wiping away what seem like masses of blood. When he returns, I tell him about the diarrhea I've had for some time and he insists that I get a CAT scan.

"Maybe I should wait for the biopsy results and if they are okay. . . ."

"You'll need the CAT scan anyway," he interrupts. I don't want a CAT scan. The dye can be bad for my kidneys. I have a history of elevated creatinine levels that show that the kidneys are not doing their job, and all that radiation is more poison in my body that can cause cancer. This will be my fourth CAT scan in a year.

I had come into to the Cancer Center full of confidence and leave full of dread. The biopsy results won't be ready for three days. For three days, chemo scenarios race through my mind, visions of sickness, weakness, and exhaustion. I have nightmares of being hospitalized. Neena is scheduled for knee replacement surgery next week, and I am scheduled for nursemaid duty during her long slow process of recovery. How will we manage if I am demolished by chemo again?

I call the nurse (Karen, not Ann, who is on vacation) on the third day for the biopsy results and get voice mail. When I call later, I'm told she is in clinic. Eventually she calls back.

"Dr. Rodriguez has had a family emergency so he has not seen the results," she says. I'm thinking, stalling tactic, but then she adds that there is no dysplasia, only granulation, no sign of a malignancy. I practically collapse with relief. Another reprieve. Another reminder that I will never be free from fear.

I had thought I had finally come to closure, that I was ready to end this journal, but I had to have a biopsy and now I need a CAT scan. I feel haunted. The devils of this disease don't cease their demonic dances.

THE DOCTOR IS IN

Unlike last year's rainy fall, we've had an autumn full of sunshine, but Indian summer never lasts, and now the cold Lake Michigan winds bend the bare branches of the trees. I put off making the CAT scan appointment, because I want to talk to Rodriguez about it again. I am getting more stomachaches, but they are exactly at my belly button, where my hernia bulges. When I call, Ann tells me Rodriguez is out for the week because his father died.

Neena has had surgery for a knee replacement, so I am running to the hospital and then to the rehab center everyday for the next weeks and put off making the CAT scan appointment. How will I be able to take care of Neena if I am zonked from chemo?

After several weeks, I call Rodriguez again. He talks me into the CAT scan with some irritation in his voice, "We've been over this before."

I've sent him a condolence card, but I say anyway, "I'm so sorry your father died."

"I never realized how hard the loss of a parent would be," he replies.

"Was he sick?"

"He had two kinds of cancer and was very sick for the last year."

"I'm so sorry." How awful it must be for an oncologist to lose a parent to cancer. I wonder if he thought he should have saved him. "How's your mother doing?"

"She's doing okay. Women are much stronger than men."

"I hope your family is getting lots of support."

"We're a large family. There's lots of love. It's a powerful experience. I've grown through this."

"I'm sure you'd rather have your father here though."

"Oh yes. We were very close."

I appreciate his speaking so personally with me. I like that about him, that he is accessible emotionally, unlike so many doctors who wall themselves off from their patients. Several days later when I call Ann to tell her the date of my CAT scan, she thanks me for the condolence card I sent, saying that it came to her and she gave it to Dr. Rodriguez and that he appreciated it.

SUPPORT GROUP, NOVEMBER

A women's center is starting a support group for women who have recently completed cancer treatment. Because I believe other cancer survivors can provide understanding and wisdom in ways that those without similar experience cannot, I join. The two leaders are young women who have not had cancer. At the first session, Dolores, the one with a high-pitched voice, speaks about how people have changed their lives for the better as a result of cancer.

"Cancer is a gift," she announces.

Yeah, sure, it's a gift. Since that's what she thinks, I'll give her my gift of cancer, along with the surgery, the chemo, the radiation, the nausea, the exhaustion, the disrupted digestion, the hair loss, the neuropathy, the fear, and the dread.

Whenever someone speaks of her cancer experience, the other leader with the lower voice, Pam, gives a learned pronouncement about finding meaning in the disease or the like. I think she should encourage connections among group members instead of making herself the hub of the wheel with spokes to the members. I wish she would respond with, "Has anyone else ever experienced that?" or some other response to connect us to one another.

Ten of the twelve women in the group have had breast cancer. All but one of them have had breast reconstruction, which they discuss several sessions later. One of them brings it up, and they describe what sounds like a ghastly process of thirteen hours of surgery, painful breast expanders, and abdominal pain so severe from removal of tissue for the new breasts they couldn't get out of bed. Another woman, who had very large breasts, feels better without them, however.

"I haven't had this experience," I say, "but I imagine I would probably be like you and not have reconstruction, it sounds so awful." I ask the woman who described the surgery if she is glad she had it done, and she says yes, she now feels like her old self. Several others agree.

Although the issue of disfigurement discussed at this session does not pertain to me, at least it is personally meaningful to the others. I'm pretty disappointed with this group, but I'll give it a little more time in the hope that it might become relevant to me also.

THE MILLS OF GOD, DECEMBER

The day before my scheduled CAT scan, I teach at Northwestern all morning and visit Neena at rehab in the afternoon. Driving home, my visual field is interrupted for about 15 minutes with a shimmering aura, followed by a severe migraine headache. I've been subject to these light shows at odd times ever since I was sixteen. They used to be followed by migraine headaches, but the pain ended about thirty or forty years ago. This time a strong migraine zaps me once again, so I pop a couple of Tylenols just before Vicky picks me up to drive downtown to the Illinois Art Therapy Association annual dinner.

We're chatting away as we zoom down the expressway, but I start having difficulty finding words. It gets worse and worse. Am I having a stroke? I am trying to say "two hours" and the best I can do is "two parts." I've heard this inability to find words described, but I could never imagine it. I can think, but I can't make the words to express the thoughts.

I become nauseous. Lucky me, I get to die from a stroke instead of from cancer.

Vicky pulls off the expressway into a shopping center and calls an ambulance. I can read the street signs to tell her where to direct the ambulance, but I have to concentrate hard to say Fullerton, rather Fulton, which is where we were headed. We wait and wait. Vicky says my face is flushed. I am not confused or unaware, just wrapped in smothering wool that seals me off from others. Strangely, sitting there in Vicky's car, waiting for the ambulance, I am unafraid. By the time I am helped into the ambulance and questioned by the paramedics, I can report everything coherently. The aphasia lasted about twenty minutes.

In the emergency room, I am being rigged up to a heart monitor and questioned. I don't want to take off my clothes, so I leave on my slacks and boots but my vest and shirt come off for all the sticky attachments to the heart monitor. My usually low blood pressure has shot up to 180, and my blood platelet count is 750,000 (400,000 is the upper edge of normal). I am admitted to the hospital and Vicky accompanies me to my room on the eighth floor with a glittering view over the nighttime city out the floor-to-ceiling window. I get to practice my Spanish because my Mexican neighbor does not speak English. Her family spends the night, so I have lots of roommates. I get a windy gurney ride through the basement corridors to radiology for a brain CAT scan. It's clear, but the headache remains. Two young male residents make pronouncements, one says TIA, transient ischemic attack, or ministroke, and the other says migraine. Vicky stays until all the action is over for the evening. I never do get dinner.

I call Judith and Claire, who live nearby, in case I need them to come tomorrow to bring me a book or some other care package for a hospital stay.

"Don't let them tell you it's nothing," Judith says. "That's what they told my brother-in-law last June when he had a TIA, and in September he had a major stroke. He's practically helpless now, and he's younger than you." I don't know how I should respond to this or whatever diagnosis I will get.

Because the room is too hot to sleep, eighty-five degrees on the thermostat, I roam the corridors. This is a surgical unit, so I don't think the other patients are in any condition to walk around. The night duty staff just stare at me as I breeze by. I feel okay, different from the other patients in their beds, very different from the way I have felt during my previous hospitalizations. This is something of a lark. A kind charge nurse lets me use the computer on the wall, so at 4 AM. I am standing in the hall sending e-mails.

The next day I get a Doppler ultrasound of my carotid arteries, which are clear. The attending physician, Dr. Pearson, comes for rounds with her entourage. I like her. She explains that one plus one plus one equals three, i.e., headache and aphasia, high blood pressure, and high platelet count equal TIA. I am reminded of "The mills of the gods grind. . . ." but I can't remember the rest. I keep thinking "painfully." I tell her I will let her know when I come up with it. After Dr. Pearson has left the unit, I do remember the rest, so a nurse says she'll fax it to her office for me. All the staff are so nice here.

"Though the mills of God grind slowly, yet they grind exceedingly small" (*Retribution*, Henry Wadsworth Longfellow). Here I am almost eighty, and my life has ground down to ultimate illnesses, or as Gilda Radner said, "It's always something" (1989).

The weather has turned sharply cold, and there is snow on the ground. I am discharged free of symptoms but too fearful of getting a stroke to be at my house alone, since Neena is still in rehab, so Tony drives me to Vicky's, where I stay for two nights. She is wonderful to me.

I see Valli Stewart, my internist, who confirms the TIA diagnosis, and a neurologist, who says I've had a textbook case migraine, including the aphasia, not a TIA. The wild card is still the high platelet count that can cause clotting or bleeding, but I cannot get in to see the hematologist for two weeks.

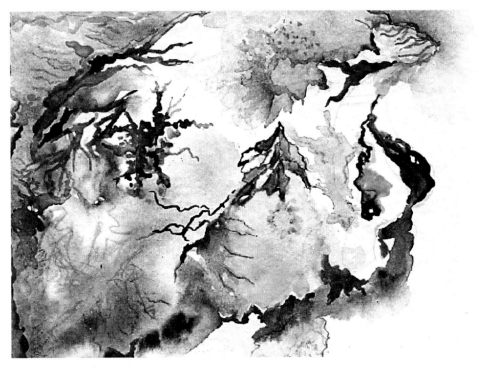

Figure 66. My brain.

I am living in layers of uncertainty. Are my digestive problems the result of cancer? Do I have a kind of blood cancer that is causing uncontrolled proliferation of platelets? Am I in danger of having a major stroke? Suppose I get a stroke and can't call for help while Neena is still staying at rehab?

Later, in a watercolor workshop with Janie Baskin at the Cancer Wellness Center, a doodle I paint becomes my brain. What is going on here? I began with a burst of yellow, perhaps some aberrant firing. Maybe there is blood vessel blockage in the red, or it all could just be normal brain activity, colorful and mysterious.

CAT SCAN, DECEMBER

The day before I bring Neena home from rehab, I go in for my rescheduled CAT scan alone. She came with me for all the others. I feel very apprehensive about the results because of all that is wrong with me, the stomachaches, the high platelets, the possible TIA. I am not happy that this will be my fifth CAT scan in thirteen months. All that radiation can cause cancer. The procedure itself has never been difficult in the past, but this time, as if in echo of my fears, the technicians have problems. I am lying on the table, and they are standing behind my head so I can't see what they are doing. A large man is putting a needle in my arm for the dye. I tell him I have small veins and he agrees. It takes him a while to get it in, which is pretty uncomfortable. The woman seems to be directing him, as though she is teaching him how to do it. They go back into the computer room, where I can hear them talking, leaving me to wait longer than usual. This is making me uneasy.

"Hello," I call to them. "Are you practicing on me?" That gets their attention. The woman comes to my side and rigs up the long arm of the machine that transports the dye to the needle.

"It doesn't hurt, does it?" she asks, checking the needle insertion in the crook of my arm.

"Yes, it hurts a little."

"It's not supposed to." She investigates the needle further. "We don't want any of the dye to leak out into your arm." She pulls the needle out and tells the guy to try the other arm.

He is apologetic and tentative, sticking me in several places before giving up. "We'll have to call in a nurse expert," the woman says.

"Can you get Gwen at the Cancer Center?" I ask. "She always gets it in on the first try."

"No, she has to stay over there."

"The people in the outpatient lab aren't any good," I say, "they always have to stick me lots of times, and if this expert is the one who's come for chemo and when I was hospitalized, she can never get it in." I don't need this along with my anxiety. We wait some more. They've already slid me in and out of the ring of the scanner a couple of times, and I'm wondering if those were wasted pictures, more radiation doses for nothing. I ask about it.

"No," the woman says, "those were scouting pictures to program the computer."

"Are the pelvis, abdomen, and chest done separately?" I might as well find out what I can while we're waiting.

"No, they're all done together. We do two scouting pictures then one of the whole area with the dye going in and another of the whole area a couple minutes after the dye injection. Then the computer slices the images into different planes." In all the past scans, I had thought they were shooting separate parts. If I weren't so antsy, I'd find the information interesting.

"When will the results be ready?" I ask.

"Today or early tomorrow morning." That means I should hear from Ann tomorrow afternoon.

The nurse expert comes and gets the needle in on the first try. Some people know how to do it and some don't, in spite of sticking dozens of veins a day. I ask her name. Tessie. I'm going to request her each time.

From the hospital I drive to visit Neena at rehab and organize her transfer home tomorrow. Ellie, Judith, and Claire will help. There are some Christmas carolers in the parlor outside Neena's room, so I go out and sing with them, then ask them to come into her room to sing to her. Fortunately, she doesn't say bah humbug in her usual anti-Christmas way but actually enjoys them. They even give her a poinsettia. All of this is good for me to get my mind off the CAT scan results.

The next day Neena's homecoming goes without a hitch, and Judith and Claire stay to visit, but my attention is poised for the ring of the phone. Rodriguez told me that if everything is alright, I won't have to come in. So if Ann says that I need an appointment, I will know that the cancer has returned. The dread tightens in my chest. The phone doesn't ring. What does that mean? That Ann's too busy and since there is no cancer, the call isn't that important? Or that because there is recurrence, she wants the doctor to call me and this is his surgery day? Finally, I call at the end of the day, but Ann has left, so I leave a message.

The next day I dread the news even more. I try to put it out of my mind and do so for brief periods. Toward late afternoon, Ann calls and apologizes for the delay.

"The doctor had to look at the pictures and talk with the radiologist."

I try to read from her voice if something is wrong. It is. Even though she is saying there is no sign of cancer.

"There is a small mass near the upper transverse colon that has not grown in the past year, but it has changed from fat to soft tissue. If it were cancer," she continues, "it would have grown or shrunk from the chemo, but it did neither. You can have it biopsied if you want to be sure, but Dr. Rodriguez says it's not worth bothering with."

I had expected to feel relieved if the scan showed no cancer, but I don't. I'm not sure why. Is it because of the nagging uncertainty about the mass? Is it because of the stomachaches and the aphasia? Is it because I've just been through too much to feel okay, and there is still the question of the increased platelets?

I wait a day and then call Rodriguez. He doesn't call back until the next day. He sounds annoyed because he told Ann to go over this with me in detail. He doesn't know what the change in tissue means and can't look anything up because he is calling from his car. The biopsy would be easy because the area is near the surface. I ask if it were him, what would he do? He says he wouldn't do anything.

His reasoning slays me: "It's a personal decision, not a medical one. If I find any cancer, I would have to start chemo. It would be better to get it later if anything shows up down the road. A day without chemo is a good day."

What am I to make of that?

HEMATOLOGY, DECEMBER

I don't expect anything conclusive from my hematology appointment two weeks later, and I don't get it. Marcia, the nurse in the vampire department, does a blood draw, saying I am very "juicy." She takes a lot and comes back with the counts quickly. The platelets are still high, 719,000; 400,000 is normal.

The hematologist Dr. Kaminer, a pleasant, slender woman, tells me that I have either primary or secondary thrombocytosis. The latter is the result of some inflammation in my body, such as cancer. The primary variety results from something wrong in the bone marrow platelet factory. The problem is that since the platelets are the clotting factor in the blood, too many of them can cause dangerous clotting, such as in the brain, causing a stroke.

"I think it's primary," she says, "but the only way to find out is by doing a bone marrow biopsy in the pelvic bone. If it's secondary, we just treat the underlying cause. If it's primary, I'll give you a kind of chemotherapy in pill form that will control the platelet proliferation."

"Uncontrolled platelet growth sounds like blood cancer," I say.

"Yes, it's a kind of cancer."

Great! Another cancer, more chemotherapy. I don't even ask about the side effects. Marcia schedules the biopsy for a month from now. I don't want to think about it, but I do look up the chemical treatment used. Hydroxyurea. It can cause leukemia!

NONSUPPORT GROUP, JANUARY

Hope springs infernal. I have now attended about eight sessions of what is supposed to be the cancer support group. At the previous meeting, I told the group that I have a possible diagnosis of a second cancer of the blood and have to get a bone marrow biopsy, but no one mentions it at this session. The scheduled topic for the evening is sex. I tell the group that I would not speak about anything as intimate as my sex life here because I don't feel that connected to others in this group. I am cut off twice, once by each of the facilitators. Pam, the one with the lower voice, urges the other women to talk about sex. Several of them say they are not having problems, and the discussion fizzles.

A few days later, Pam calls me on the phone to discuss my lack of connection with the group. I talk about being cut off by her, and she launches into an attack with big guns, saying that others in the group have complained to her about me, specifically about my remark that I would probably be like the one person in the group who chose not to have breast reconstruction. When I suggest that any reactions to my remark should be brought up in the group, she doesn't want that at all. She questions my remaining in the group.

"Is the purpose of this call to encourage me to stay in the group or to leave it?" I ask.

"It's to help you to find ways to feel more connected."

"I'll think over staying or leaving the group and let you know." I have the distinct feeling, though, that she is trying to get me to leave.

I talk it over with Neena, wondering why there is even a question in my mind about staying in the group. What I realize is that I would like so much to have the support of a group of women who are also survivors of hell. Having cancer is bad enough; I don't need the leader of a group in which I am supposed to be getting support to be battling me as well. I decide to exit, and a few days later in order to have closure, I send an e-mail to the other members saying goodbye and wishing them well.

Before I can send another e-mail to the two leaders, Pam calls again. "Things were left up in the air when we talked last, but because you have been so disruptive in the group, I think you should leave." I can hardly believe what I am hearing, but long ago I realized that the phone is not a good transmitter for a heavy discussion.

"I have already decided to do so."

"Would you like a recommendation for a therapist since you have a possible second cancer diagnosis?"

"No thank you." I am flabbergasted. I decide it is better to say as little as possible. I say goodbye and hang up.

I receive a couple e-mail replies from the group members, wishing me well. One of them says she is sorry I am leaving because she has always liked my input. She is not sure if she is getting anything out of the group either.

This whole experience is amazing to me. Here are professional counselors hired to work with cancer survivors about their most vulnerable issues. Here I am, having announced that I might even have a second cancer, but because I dare to say that the group she is running is not one in which I feel very connected, the leader cuts me off in the group, attacks me over the phone, and tells me to leave the group because I am so "disruptive." This is supposed to be a support group! How can people who are so defensive be hired to work with those who are trying to survive cancer? What kind of training could this leader have had, or lacked, that she knows so little of group process? Cancer patients get very harsh medical treatment. We don't need harsh emotional treatment as well from those hired to help us!

HAPPY BIRTHDAY

I have just turned eighty. That is so old. Many people my age are dead, but I am energetic and spry, my mind is full of ideas, can I really be this old? Neena gives me a marvelous party with about forty-five people that I help plan, provision, and set up. It's a wonderful occasion. I am fortunate to have such great friends. John and Ellen bring a sound system with a mike and speakers for the entertainment, beginning with a song they have written for me that they play on the guitar and banjo, getting everyone to join in the chorus. The singing is followed by many beautiful and funny poems, a puppet enactment by Tamara of a conversation between me and Freud with a puppet she made of me, more songs from Robinlee and her guitar and Happy Birthday in Italian from Margherita and Bart. Although I asked guests not to bring gifts, I am given adornments for my head, a beautiful hat Robinlee felted for me, a big crown Joanna made for me, and the diamond tiara I have always wanted from Sacha and Sue.

This will probably be my last big birthday bash ever, unless I live until ninety, which no longer seems very likely. Mukherjee (2010) doesn't seem to think that having cancer at an advanced age is such a bad thing. He sees cancer as a part of who we are. This condition is so intimately interwoven into our destiny that our aim should not be to rid ourselves of it but to push it into our old age. As he puts it, "It is possible that we are fatally conjoined to this ancient illness, forced to play its cat-and-mouse game for the foreseeable future of our species. But if cancer deaths can be prevented before old age, if the terrifying game of treatment, resistance, recurrence, and more treatment can be stretched out longer and longer, then it will transform the way we imagine this ancient illness. Given what we know about cancer, even this would represent a technological victory unlike any other in our history. It would be a victory over our own inevitability—a victory over our genomes" (Mukherjee, 2010). In this sense, at eighty my life in Cancer Land is more or less timely.

TO BIOPSY OR NOT TO BIOPSY

Aside from all the hoopla of my birthday, what I am up to is researching this blood platelet problem. I scour the Web and make the mistake of watching a video of the bone marrow biopsy procedure. It's like taking a core sample from the earth or the ice in Antarctica, drilling deep to extract a core whose layers can show a history. In my case, it will be a core of marrow from the back of the hip bone for a history of blood platelet development. The video doctor pushes and pushes to get the needle, that's as thick as a pencil, deep into the bone.

Another thing, it's usually done if the platelet count is 750,000 to 1 million. Mine was less, 719,000 at the last count. Why not continue monitoring, why not continue taking iron pills since anemia can cause this, why not continue a double dose of aspirin, suggested by the neurologist to prevent clotting? So I am going in to see the doctor, who is prepared to do the biopsy, with all my questions and objections.

The Kellogg Cancer Center parking lot is full. Cancer is big business. I park illegally in one of the striped areas between the handicapped places. Gwen, who usually draws my blood at the Cancer Center, does so efficiently as always. I am ushered into a large, brightly lit room with a bed. At first I don't see any other place to sit. The aide says that shortly I will be on the bed anyway.

"Maybe not," I say as I notice a chair in the corner. I put down my stuff and go out to the waiting room to get Neena. Dr. Kaminer comes in followed by two white-coated young women. Her cell rings and she goes out of the room to answer it. Neena asks the young women if they are residents. They are. I ask them about the procedure, figuring I may get more complete information from them than from the doctor.

"We've done three this morning and everyone walked off the table," one says.

"No one cried," the other adds.

Dr. Kaminer returns.

"We may have a fight," I tell her, "so I've brought my second." I introduce her to Neena.

"I've brought my backups, too," she says, introducing the residents. We're all very jovial. I ask questions. She answers.

"I called Dr. Rodriguez and he said your last CAT scan shows that you are stable now. So it doesn't look as though you have secondary thrombocytosis caused by the cancer. He also said he was very impressed with your art book you showed him." I am amazed he even remembered it. I brought my altered book into an appointment nine months ago. "Since you are over sixty and had what may have been a TIA ministroke, treatment would be advisable. But I wouldn't want to put you on chemotherapy without being sure it is primary thrombocytosis, caused by a bone marrow abnormality, and the only way to be sure is the bone marrow biopsy." She shakes her head when I ask about other treatments, such as blood thinners. "They're riskier than the hydroxyurea we would use." She directs one of the residents to get a printout about the medication and tells me that its chance of causing leukemia is rare and would occur only in ten or fifteen years. I'd be dead by then anyway. "The chemo you've had, Carboplatin and Taxol, are more likely to cause it."

"Would I need to be on it the rest of my life?" She nods.

An aide comes in and hands Kaminer a sheet of paper.

"You're platelet count is 681,000," she says, "and there are abnormal cells."

"Isn't that a good sign, that it's lower?" I ask.

"It's still the same ballpark as the 719,000 last time." She looks at her watch. "We're running out of time to do the procedure."

"If it were me, I'd get the biopsy," Neena says. "I'd want to know. That's why I'm a scientist. But that's just me. I have a different personality from yours."

For some crazy reason, I am determined to lower my platelets on my own by sheer force of my own will plus the iron I am taking for borderline anemia that can cause increased platelets. The neurologist had recommended a double dose of the aspirin I was taking already to reduce the risk of a stroke. "Let's wait," I say. "Can you just monitor it for a while longer?"

"That's not my first recommendation, but I can live with that. We'll check it again in six weeks." She leaves with her entourage. I put on my coat and glance at the paper on hydroxyurea. Side effects: lowered white and red blood cells. In other words, fatigue and suppressed immune system. Avoid crowds, the paper directs. No theater, no planes, no large parties, avoidance of people with colds. It states that side effects would cease once treatment is over. Mine would never be over.

I stop to make an appointment for six weeks from now at the reception desk in the large attractive waiting room with its high ceiling, plants, and uniformed door woman who greets those coming and going. I say goodbye and leave that sod house of sorrows.

MARROW

A few days later, I go to a hypnosis workshop at the Cancer Wellness Center. Harry, the presenter, seems like a nice, gentle sort of guy, but he is talking too long. He mentions some Buddhist monks

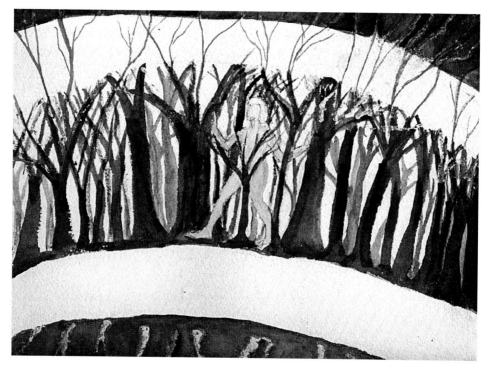

Figure 67. Bone marrow.

who could control their bodies through self-hypnosis and make them warm while out in the snow. They poured water on one another, and steam rose. Eventually he gets to what I came for, the hypnosis itself. I close my eyes, lie back in the chair, and breathe. I am relaxed, sometimes hearing Harry's words and sometimes not. Maybe I am in a trance. I visualize my bone marrow. I see a dark thicket. It becomes a forest. I imagine myself in the midst of it, bringing healing to it so that only healthy blood cells will be formed. If the monks could control physiological processes, maybe I can too.

When I get home, I greet Neena hastily in my rush to paint the visualization. I like the image and keep returning to it both with my brush and afterwards in my mind's eye. At the same time that I am trying to do the metaphysical, control my platelet production of which I am not even aware, the focus on my bone marrow shrinks my denial. I have to admit to myself that a high platelet count most likely signals either a return of my cancer or a kind of blood cancer that can lead to a stroke and that there is a strong possibility I will have to be on chemotherapy for the rest of my life. I decide that if my platelet count is still high in three weeks when I see Rodriguez, I won't wait three weeks more for my appointment with Kaminer to schedule a bone marrow biopsy.

I gaze at my painting of the woman making her way through the dense forest of blood-red trees sealed in white bone, and once again I feel the love for painting that transforms this nightmare into something more like a strange dream.

"MY FUNNY VALENTINE"

When I see Rodgriguez for my three-month checkup, all is well, except for my platelets, which are still high, 661,000, a little lower than last time but not much. He says that if my stomachaches were due to cancer, they would be persistent, increasing in intensity, rather than intermittent as they are now. That is a huge relief. One doubt down. I tell him about this book, that I am almost ready to send it off to the publisher and that he plays a major part throughout.

We talk about the possible TIA and the bone marrow biopsy. He shakes his head. "You don't want to get a stroke. You'll become a different person. You're a creative individual." He shakes his head again and sighs. "Get the bone marrow biopsy." I make an appointment for Valentine's Day.

Arriving for the biopsy, I give Dr. Kaminer a peace offering, a couple of heart decorations from the party and some heart-shaped cookies. No residents this time, so I don't have to worry if she is turning the procedure over to a resident to get some practice. I am lying on my stomach on the bed so I can't see what's happening, but I can feel it. She wipes an area of my back just below the waist to the right of my spine, the iliac crest of the pelvic bone. She is telling me about a book she just finished, saying she thinks it might interest me. It is set on a mental ward and is about an artist who became a psychiatrist because he didn't think his art was good enough. I like the distraction of the story.

"I've reached the bone," she says about the stinging anesthesia needle. I imagine it long. Then she pokes around, saying, "I'm trying to find the spot I anesthetized." I wonder why she didn't mark it. Where she's poking hurts. Maybe she won't find it. I'm not sure if she's got it, but since I'm waffling, she starts inserting, drilling into me, as I visualize it. It hurts. I want another story, but I don't want Kaminer to be distracted so I call to Neena, who comes closer and starts what is supposed to be a story.

"We worked with animals and one of the students was being sadistic to a dog. . . ."

"No," I yell. "I don't want sadism. Tell me something pleasant." I'm shouting ouch too much to hear anything anyway.

"Now it's going to feel like a kick in the gut," Kaminer says. I brace myself for what is probably the aspiration of the marrow. It isn't as bad as I expect. She's finished. She'll call me in two days with the results.

THE MARROW OF THE MATTER, FEBRUARY

My cancer destiny continues to unfold in leaves of freedom and capture. Ann calls to tell me that my Pap test showed only changes resulting from radiation and chemotherapy, no malignancies: "Negative for intraepithelial lesion/malignancy (NIL/M). Reactive cellular changes associated with therapy (radiation and/or chemotherapy)," the report reads on the computer copy she e-mails me. So that part of my body is safe for now.

Today I await Dr. Kaminer's call to learn about my blood. I'll find out if I have a kind of blood cancer that will keep me on chemo for the rest of my life to stave off a stroke. This evening we will meet Judith and Claire for dinner and the opera. Tomorrow I will do my taxes and read material for the novel-writing group, and in two weeks we will go to Florida to end the winter. I have been invited to give several presentations on my cancer art when I return. I will teach my spring course at Northwestern. In other words, my life will continue, for a while anyway.

I sort out bills and tax statements, a mindless activity, waiting for the phone to ring. I take deep breaths. I imagine feeling chemo fatigue for the rest of my life. I fantasize happy relief when Kaminer tells me I don't have primary thrombocytosis. I banish that fantasy and warn myself to prepare for the worst, what may be a long slow death.

The phone rings. At first Kaminer doesn't seem to know what to say. Alarms go off in my head. She talks about white cells that are not right, suspicious I guess. It's all a jumble. I don't have primary thrombocytosis, but the white cell problem could be linked to lymphoma, but the CAT scan didn't show anything. The bottom line, she says, is that we will do nothing now. I ask her to explain what is going on, what's causing the increase in platelets. She doesn't know. I ask if their increase could be related to the abnormal leucocytes, and she says yes, they could be related to lymphoma. We will have to continue monitoring my blood count, once every three months, and I should see her again in six. Is this a reprieve, a stay of execution? All these days without chemo will be good days. But now dread shows yet another new face, abnormal leucocytes, lymphoma?

Since what Kaminer says is so confusing, I am hoping that the written report will be more clarifying. Neena will be able to explain unfamiliar terms. Kaminer hasn't gotten it yet. I wait a day and send an e-mail to remind her to send it. She e-mails back that it is not yet finalized. I keep checking North Shore Connect, the e-mail service where I can communicate with my doctors and get my test results. It isn't there. I had the biopsy Monday morning. Kaminer called on Wednesday. Now it is Friday evening and Neena and I are about to leave for the theater. I open my e-mail one more time, and there it is.

The biopsy report covers three pages, single spaced. There are many acronyms, numbers, and percentages. There are lots of words I don't recognize, but among them are "leukemia" and "lymphoma." In a state of shock, I leave for the play. I drive, because Neena can no longer drive at night. I concentrate hard on the road. In the theater, my mind wanders from the play. When we get home, I print out the report for Neena and send Kaminer an e-mail, asking her to explain the report. Since it is Friday night, I probably won't hear anything over the weekend so I will have to endure this anxiety tightness in my chest until next week. The biopsy was a search for wayward blood platelet origins, but it has revealed aberrant white cells as well. Cancer is full of unexpected anguish. I had been happy. I thought I had been given back my life, for another three months anyway, but now, the crab clutches tighter.

After a weekend of anxiety and depression, I call Kaminer on Monday morning. She calls back Monday afternoon. When I ask her to explain the biopsy report, she says it was not meant for a layperson's eyes. There is only a "suspicion" of essential thrombocytosis, so I don't need chemotherapy now, we will just watch it. The leukemia could cause the platelet increase, but in itself it is not an issue. If it were a problem, enlarged lymph nodes or an enlarged spleen would have shown up on my CAT scan.

"You could have the leukemia for decades. If we hadn't done the bone marrow biopsy, you wouldn't even have known you have it," Kaminer says. "What is the word I want? Inconsequential. The results are inconsequential." I could have done without the weekend of unnecessary anguish.

Kaminer is saying what I had determined before the biopsy, that since the platelets were not that high, we should just monitor my blood count. The doctors want to investigate my insides with CAT scans and biopsies. Maybe I can be free of them for a while, at least until I get another investigation.

ENDING

I am feeling well. I am eighty years old and full of life. The well-being I took for granted for most of my life is now a precious gift, but I live in Cancer Land, a city of shadows. Demons lurk around every corner. I've never seen one of them, but my doctors have. Sometimes I wonder where I would be now if I'd never seen a doctor.

"Dead," Rodriguez says.

What is this thing called cancer anyway, if not overly active cells, eager to live and proliferate? They just keep growing and surviving, pushing their less-aggressive, mortal cousins out of the way. They are the part of us that refuses to die. So we approach them with the deadliest weapons we can find, scalpels, radioactivity, poisons. Never mind that our arsenals lay waste our well-behaved cells too. Cancer treatment often hinges on how much devastation the patient can stand. Sometimes not enough. Radiation and some chemotherapies generate new cancers. The treatment can be so effective that it not only kills the cancer cells, it kills the patient as well.

In future generations, our progeny may understand how and why cells mutate into promiscuous rogues who refuse to stay in line. Perhaps they will find ways to induce them to behave, rather than relying on weapons of mass destruction as we do today. We may even learn something about extending life from them. I wonder if our descendents will view this thing called cancer differently from our death dread. Most likely they will look upon today's cancer treatments as primitive, if not barbaric.

So what does an eighty-year-old girl who has been granted a reprieve from cancer do today? She lives her life. She finishes this journal and sends her book to the publisher; she turns her attention to writing her novel; she makes sketches for the large painting she is planning about cancer; she does her taxes; she goes to Florida to finish off winter in the sun rather than in the snow. She hopes her doctors know what they are doing. She has to admit that she harbors some degree of admiration for those feisty cancer cells that won't stay put.

In ending this journal, I have come to realize that some of us cancer survivors must live with our cancers all the rest of our lives. Cancer Land is our permanent residence. Life *In the Clutch of the Crab* prickles with dread.

Perhaps the ending is that there is no ending.

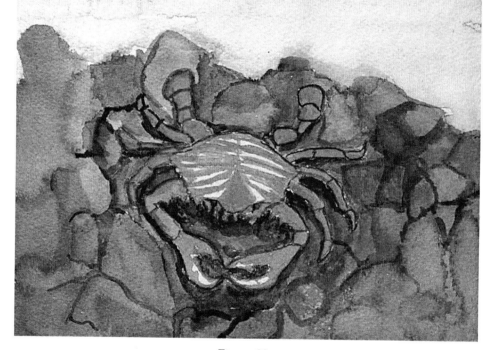

Figure 68.

5

CANCER LAND:
AN ALTERED BOOK FOR AN ALTERED LIFE

Although images are static, a book is sequential. It can tell a story. A book seemed to me to be the perfect container for images of my experience. I was not feeling well midway in my chemotherapy and radiation treatment, but I did not want to miss the opportunity to attend an Altered Book Workshop being held at the Cancer Wellness Center. I had never tried making altered books, and I was only vaguely aware of them as an art form from an exhibit I had seen many years before. The more complicated book arts in the exhibit were not what I had in mind. I simply wanted to tell my story in images.

An altered book is a mixed media artwork that changes a book from its original form by altering its appearance and/or meaning. Material may be added by drawing, painting, gluing, tying, and stitching and subtracted by cutting, tearing, or burning. The shape of pages or of the entire book may be changed. The original text may be utilized or covered over or cut out in whole or part.

There were only four of us in the workshop, but the teacher, Janie Baskin, was enthusiastic, and she had brought lots of materials. From the books that she supplied for us to alter, I selected one whose size and shape I liked, as well as the picture of the young woman on the cover (which I later replaced with another image because the woman was too different from me). Janie suggested subjects for our books, such as the seasons, travel, animals, love, landscapes, and many more. When she asked me what my subject would be, I said, "Cancer." That was not on her long list.

A book has shape and heft. I knew from the start that I wanted to sculpt it in some way. My first thought was a black hole, the black hole my life had fallen into. I would bore it through a clump of pages.

In examples of altered books Janie had made, I saw pockets with contents that could slide in and out, an image on a page peeking through the hole of the page in front of it, and small pages that only partially covered others. In other words, altered books can become interactive as the reader lifts a covering or pulls something out of a pocket. I liked that aspect. It offers surprise, not unlike pop-up books that I have loved since childhood.

Janie's first instruction was for us to tear out a number of pages throughout the book, because what we would glue in would add to the bulk so that the book wouldn't close with all its original pages. Next she showed us how to make pockets. I liked the idea of tucking things away so that they could not be seen unless pulled out. Some parts of my experience needed to be hidden. I perused the papers she had brought. Many were brightly colored with designs of flowers, birds, and other pretty things. I bypassed these and chose a sheet that looked like camouflage and another of leopard spots. The first pocket was to be slanted. I wasn't sure where to put it in the book since I was telling a story and didn't know where it would fall in the sequence, so the placement was random, in the middle somewhere. All I knew at that time about the book's sequence was that I would have to leave a clump of pages for my black hole that would bore through many layers, becoming smaller and smaller.

What follows are discussions of my processes in creating the altered book. The pictures that are referenced below are reproduced in full color on the enclosed CD at the back of this book.

CD 1: Cancer Land: An Altered Book for an Altered Life

CD 2: Janie had brought pictures of objects, and I chose what looked like Hamlet holding Yoric's skull and buried it in a pocket of camouflage paper. My first image was of hidden death. At home, I decided that the Hamlet page needed something more, so I added a painting I had made of birds on the beach. I don't know why. Maybe I wanted some life in it, the birds, the beach, the sea. I was already familiar with scanning my paintings into my computer and printing them in a reduced size from having done so on greeting cards and silk scarves I made. Throughout my altered book, I utilized this technique.

CDs 3, 4: I did not find an object for my second, horizontal leopard pocket until I got home. It became a small book of the leopard's strength. As is often the case in my artwork, the materials dictated the content, although clearly, my choice of materials was not random.

At home, I became absorbed in making my altered book, despite often feeling too sick to gather the materials I needed, so that I used those I had already spread out on my table: paint and brushes, many different papers, glue, ribbons, and eventually my hair. I painted pictures in watercolors that found their way into my book via the computer process. Because I frequently felt ill while I was creating them, some of the pages are sloppy, particularly their titles that I usually added at the end when I was exhausted. Because of my limited energy, I used simple materials and finished many of the pages in single sessions. Although sometimes I worked on the pages in sequence, often I skipped around. But I tried to leave blank pages to fill later so that the book would be in the chronological order of my experience.

Except for the first two pictures that I made at the Altered Book Workshop, the pages are presented here in the book's sequence, so that you can view them as if you were reading the book, rather than in the order in which I made them. Because this is a twice-told tale in words and in images, there is some repetition of what I wrote about creating some of the pages in the written journal.

CD 5: I used ribbons to cover the book's original title and author on both the spine and the book's cover, pasting in my own title and name. For a long time I left the image of the dark-haired young woman from the original. I liked her, but after working on the book a while, I realized I couldn't use her. She was just too much un-me. By then, I was wearing a wig with long white hair, made from my own hair that I had cut for that purpose before it all fell out. I have a Japanese doll holding a wig of long white hair that I thought would serve the purpose, so I photographed her and used the print for the cover. The Japanese geisha seemed emblematic of the merely decorative value of women, and since my cancer had been lodged in my uterus, it was clearly a woman's disease. From the book I hung a black-beaded ninja holding a box of crayons that was made by an art therapy student and given to me by my former student Vicky.

CD 6: As is evident from this photo, the finished book is too bulky, too full. It is not neat as are the examples Janie showed us of books she had made. Even though I had torn out a number of the book's original pages, as Janie instructed, I didn't realize how thick the glued pages would be. I don't mind that my book is not a nice neat compendium. My experience was not neat either. A book that does not close properly, that is too full, seems representative of my life.

Collages of magazine images were easier than drawing when I felt particularly bad, as art therapists know from our work with clients. More recently, I have painted pictures to replace some of them for the published version of the book, because I have no idea from what publications I got some of the pictures.

CD 7: The title page is an example of the altering I did. I had chosen a picture of cancer's astrological sign, in this case red crabs from our visit to the Galapagos Islands, probably from a travel brochure, and left the word "becoming" from the book's original title page. Subsequently, I painted crabs to cover the brochure image.

CD 8: Later I replaced my crude printing with computerized printing.

CD 9: And later still, I painted a picture of a red crab on dark rocks, inspired by the original travel photo.

CD 10: Another sheet of paper that I had taken from Janie's supply reminded me of cells. I used it for the first page and began the book with the quote from my internist, "At seventy-eight, you don't need anymore Pap tests, but . . ."

CD 11: The cell paper continues onto the next page as does the internist's message, "It showed suspicious cells!" The crabs wander onto the facing page, along with some wild cells.

CD 12: The next two pages continue the introductory material. There is a small crab in the corner and orange labels announcing "Property of Harriet Wadeson." They form the opening page of a small book made from printed pages of the original book.

CD 13: The first page says, "An Altered Book For . . ."

CD 14: "An Altered Life!" is written on the next page.

CD 15: The facing page is covered with an orange veil. Beneath it is a painting of Muslim women with covered faces (another reduced painting I'd made) with the title "A WOMAN'S WORLD." Uterine cancer is a woman's disease. Women's reproductive systems, along with their diseases, have long been veiled.

CD 16: Door County was a tranquil respite before the onslaught of diagnosis and treatment.

CD 17: Then the treatment begins. Woozy from chemo, I banged my shin against a table leg and it bled like crazy. I was grabbing paper napkins off the table to mop up the blood, when it occurred to me that the blotchy napkins might be useful. So in they went to the book's pages on my hysterectomy, surrounding a picture of the operation. (Artists collect the strangest objects for their work.)

CD 18: During surgery, cancer cells were found in my abdominal cavity and the omentum, a fatty layer that covers the small intestine. It had spread. I had stage III cancer. The news was devastating to me. I would need chemotherapy and radiation. What was my body doing? I used a painting of DNA I had made to represent the wild growth of cancer that results from damaged DNA and cut a copy of it into a book within the book to reveal the news.

CD 19: Inside, I glued crabs, diseased cells, and a photo of a red screaming mask I had made. I hoped it depicted my anguish.

CD 20: The back of the DNA book.

CD 21: Although I had placed the camouflaged Hamlet death pages toward the middle of the book at the workshop when I first started, I was now able to tear out the intervening pages of the original book so the death pages come next, which felt appropriate for the ultimate fear of cancer metastases. It needed something more, so later I glued on the painting of the birds on the beach. They add some life.

CD 22: On the page following are dark clouds that were now covering my life. I hadn't meant the mountains to look like breasts.

CD 23: The many people who have been supportive were very important to me during my treatment. "Friends bring food . . ." is the title of pages crowded with lots of dishes. I made some of the objects on this and other pages pop out by gluing them onto paper pedestals, but the three-dimensional aspect of the pictures does not show in the reproductions.

CD 24: "Friends bring food . . ." is followed by ". . . and flowers" on the next pages. I added a reduction of my painting of "Shattered Tulips."

CD 25: "Shattered Tulips," flowers brought to me by Vicky that became interesting to me for a painting when they began to fall apart. Identification?

CD 26: A plant Helen brought. I enjoyed showing her the painting the next time she visited. In addition to visits from friends, colleagues, and students, I received many messages from people out of town, some I didn't even know, who knew me from my books and presentations. Art therapy students from four different schools sent drawings and paintings. Some of these messages and pictures went into the book. That so many were praying for me and sending me their good wishes was immensely important to me. It is in times like this that we benefit from the support from others. I felt cared about by so many people.

CD 27: While I was recovering from surgery, on an impulse, my daughter Lisa decided to spend her birthday with me, which was a big deal for her and her husband Mark to get away, and Lisa is afraid of flying, which made it an extra effort for her. I included a picture from their visit.

CD 28: Although we went out for a fancy birthday dinner, I had trouble eating it. I not only lost parts of my body in surgery, I lost my appetite as well, so I put that on the facing page.

CD 29: The next pages herald the beginning of chemotherapy. I brought oil pastels to my first chemo session and drew my hand with all the tape and tubes attached and the pole holding the bags of infusion. For the book, however, I wanted to add something about how I felt. I pasted on messy, crinkled brown paper and a photo of a mask I had made that to me looks horror struck.

CD 30: A few days later, I painted blue chemicals zapping the cancer and blood cells, with new blood cells replacing them. The cancer cells are little orange crabs, and the blood cells are red, white, and yellow for the platelets. I mounted the painting on deep blue shiny paper, the color I used for the killing chemicals. The picture ended up looking more delicate than I expected.

CD 31: I had to take lots of medications, so in went pills with cells that are being affected by them.

CD 32: I didn't know how to represent the nausea and the all-over sick feeling I had from chemo. I settled for wooziness that I represented by painting a picture of buildings on the water to suggest seasickness as they are superimposed on each other in a wobbly way so that the picture doesn't quite cohere.

CD 33: Chemo brain was easier. I had brought home swirly paper from Janie's supply, and I cut out eyeballs from the cell-like paper to put into eyes made from transparent yellow cellophane. I hope the image conveys confusion.

CD 34: Peripheral neuropathy became another side effect. I cut my paintings of cells into hands and feet and added red glitter coming out of them to show their constant tingling. A photo of a mask I'd made of a very pained face is in their midst. The peripheral neuropathy persists to this day.

CD 35: Hair became an important part of my book, partly because I had so much of it. My long white hair was probably my most distinguishing feature. For some time, I had saved the hair from haircuts and from my brush to use on masks I made, so I had plenty of it around to include in the book. I glued in an old picture of myself that shows up my long hair and opposite a picture taken right after having it cut for a wig to be made from it. Between them I pasted in some of my actual hair.

CD 36: I am hidden away in an envelope after most of my hair had fallen out (I never took a picture of myself completely bald) and, opposite, wearing the wig made from my hair. The wigmaker had straightened it to make weaving in the hairs one by one easier, so it didn't really look like my hair after all. I felt like an imposter wearing it.

CD 37: More cells appear, some of them sort of messed up, with the book's original text showing through. I can't explain this image exactly, but it is something about the continuing theme of my cells growing, sometimes healthfully and sometimes destructively. I think the text represents my ongoing life.

CD 38: In midsummer, my daughter Lisa and her husband Mark visited us in Door County, WI. I usually spend the summer there and wasn't sure I would feel well enough to make it, but Lisa's planned visit with us there was a strong motivation. I glued in a reduction of a painting of the view of Ellison Bay from our living room.

CD 39: By then, I was wearing a hat all the time. Lisa bought me the fur hat in the picture of Lisa, Neena, and me at a traditional Wisconsin fish boil. Lisa and Mark enjoyed the great white fish and the flames shooting high above the restaurant's roof.

CD 40: Back to the hospital, "My Docs" cover the next pages, the integrative medicine doctor, Dr. Leslie Mendoza-Temple, whom I saw several times, on the left and Dr. Gustavo Rodriguez, my oncologist who treated me throughout, on the right. They are both wise and kind. I have appreciated their care.

CD 41: In chemo again, I requested that the music therapist visit me. When she asked what I wanted to do, I said I wanted to be entertained. She brought her guitar and we sang together. I decided to make up chemo words to the songs. I sang them and she wrote them down and later typed them up and sent them to me, where they are now pasted in the book and tucked in a pocket.

CD 42: At my next chemo treatment, I was partially knocked out but awake enough to know I had restless legs. I couldn't stop moving them. Then I got restless everything else and kept jumping up out of my chair, sitting in another chair, jumping up, and coming back to the first one. A couple of nurses yelled at me to stay still because I would interfere with the chemo flow. I didn't even answer them. Next I woke up in a bed. I didn't remember being moved. I kept trying to push down the sides so I could escape. Later I was told that in the bed my legs looked as though I was running. When they finally unhooked me, the nurse said I was there an extra hour because my moving had compressed the tube, stopping the chemo flow.

CD 43: Radiation was a horrible experience that felt like medieval torture. Various instruments were shoved roughly into my lower orifices, and I was wheeled with them in place from one freezing room to another and then left by myself and told not to move for half an hour while I waited on the table for the radiologist and then another half hour alone because I was radioactive while a beeping machine irradiated my insides. I didn't know how to depict this horror so I drew a sort of abstract, because the reality would have been too ghastly to draw. On the left is the radiation machine and above it my hospital ID bracelet. I felt like little more than a bar code to the rough radiologist. On the right, the lower orange lines are my legs and between them the pod that was stuffed inside me to blast the radiation into me. It is connected to the machine and around it are waves of radioactivity. Red glitter surrounds the red pod, showing that it can burn. I had to have three of these treatments.

CD 44: I became weak from dehydration, as represented by the desert, and had to go to the hospital for rehydration twice. Once again, I got the drip for several hours. As usual, I was stuck a number of times because the technicians had difficulty finding a vein.

CD 45: Fortunately, my strong leopard was already on the next pages.

CD 46: I had filled more than half of the book, and I needed a lot of pages for the black hole my life had fallen into, so this was the place to start burrowing. As an introduction, I painted a picture from a magazine photo of a sinkhole in a third-world country that had fallen in.

CD 47: Then I started cutting through a number of the next pages and painted the rim of the hole black on all of them. On the first page I painted swirling autumn colors and glued on red leaves I had shellacked. I had spent the whole summer in treatment and now it was fall.

CD 48: I wanted to give the impression of the hole sucking in what was around it, so on the next page I painted cooler colors along with the glitter of life pulled into it. An autumn leaf shows through, its brightness contrasting with the dark hole.

CD 49: One of the more obvious things that had gone down the hole was my hair, so I glued on some of it I had saved from my brush when it was long and added photos of myself wearing the hats that covered my head constantly all during the fall. I no longer had eyebrows or eyelashes either. The knitted caps, donated to the Cancer Wellness Center by knitting groups, each came with a message pinned to it, so I included them as well. On the left, is a head scarf my daughter-in-law Carin knitted for me, and at lower right is my wig on the stand I had painted for it.

CD 50: Cancer the Crab looms large on the next pages. I was hoping to get rid of it, but it was still dominating my life.

CD 51: Once again there are cells, this time with the message "The FUTURE Is NOW!" inspired by a photo from a medical magazine. I think the message can be read several ways, that the present misery is what my future will be, or more hopefully that I must be positive now for a healthy future. The green cells look healthy, so I prefer to read it that way.

CD 52: As I approached the end of treatment, I became sicker and sicker from the chemo. It has a cumulative effect. I had to be hospitalized for several days and have a culture grown for a suspected infection, the greatest danger for chemo patients with their suppressed immune systems. I also had to be hydrated again. The technicians couldn't get the infusion to flow and kept sticking me with the insertion needle. The unit was short staffed so I couldn't get the help I needed to go to the bathroom while attached to the IV pole. I felt tethered to the bed and painted myself that way. One night, I had to climb over the side railings of the bed, painted very prominently in the picture, because no nurse or assistant came when I called for help to get to the bathroom. When I look at this picture, I'm brought back to the misery of what was a very low point in my entire experience of cancer.

CD 53: I had planned to go to Door County for the beautiful October colors, but I was too sick to travel. I gathered autumn leaves anyway that I shellacked and glued into the book. The hole through the pages is much smaller now.

CD 54: Finally, my treatment was finished, "The End of the Summer of My Discontent," signified by an autumn painting on the last pages of the hole. This painting looks to me like a celebration of autumn. The end of chemo was certainly cause for celebration.

CD 55: I couldn't finish the book until I got the results from my CAT scan to determine if the chemo had eliminated the cancer. "CAT SCAN," shows an alert large feline, no pussycat here.

CD 56: Facing the cat are the mixed results, exuberance that there are no tumors, with petals of pain and anxiety leaving me, and beneath it, a snake and crabs in the grass and a bloody spot on the water with roots under the sea to represent the suspicious area that could be just an enlarged lymph node or it could be cancer. I wouldn't know until my next CAT scan three months later.

While I was living in the black hole, I was making pictures of what I wanted to do when I got out of it, a vision of a life beyond patienthood. On days when I felt sick, I distracted myself by creating images of what then felt like a very distant future, the end of the long, dark tunnel. I glued these in near the end of the book.

CD 57: The first picture is a painting I'd made of a young woman nude. It's not that I expected my body to look like that again, but I hoped I would feel good about it, that it would seem healthy and trustworthy to me once more. The woman is a bit tentative, dipping her toe in the water, maybe dipping into life again. She seems to be looking out over the water, perhaps wondering what is out there for her.

CDs 58, 59: The next pages are paintings of travel, to exotic Africa and to Door County.

CD 60: I wanted to attend theatrical productions of drama, music, and dance. I missed travel and theater during chemo when I was avoiding crowds by staying away from theaters and planes because my immune system was suppressed. I sprinkled the picture with sequins to make it festive.

CD 61: With more energy, I wanted to be outside and to enjoy nature. The purple butterfly pops out. The butterfly is such an intriguing creature. It's sluggish as a caterpillar, then mysterious as a chrysalis, turning to liquid to reform into the amazingly delicate and colorful creature that lights upon the flowers. Its wings are like flying flower petals.

CD 62: I wanted to see more of the people important to me, Neena, my children and their spouses, grandchildren, and my brother. When I was able to travel again, among my first trips were to the East Coast to see my children and to the West Coast to see my son and his family. Shortly afterwards, my brother and his wife came to visit me. I created these pages when I was feeling particularly bad. They were easy to make just by cutting and gluing. I have included one of them here, of my son and grandchildren.

CD 63: I needed to include my parents, long deceased, for reasons I don't understand. I think it was something about making my life whole. The picture I used is the last one taken of the four of us. I added a feather, for flight perhaps. I had found a dead monarch butterfly and attached it with surgical tape for beauty, transformation, and change. Monarchs migrate thousands of miles following the flight paths of ancestors they have never known.

CD 64: On my parents' page is a message of hope. As I go forward, I take with me the trails of ancestors.

CD 65: I thought my beginnings were a fitting ending until Thanksgiving, when my son and family visited. Instead of my fore-bears, I decided to end with my descendants, my grandchildren. I wanted to give thanks. Shortly before Thanksgiving, I had been able to travel for the first time and present a paper at the AATA Annual Conference. Being able to travel again was a significant milestone for me, so I included it on the facing page.

CD 66: At Thanksgiving, I promised my granddaughter Michaela that I would attend her high school graduation in June. I had no idea whe-ther I would be in treatment again by then or be cancer free and feel-ing well. So when I was able to travel to California six months later, the graduation of a grandchild seemed even more fitting for an end-ing. I had left a black end page blank, so I had one last page to use. Eight months after finishing chemo, I was feeling well with my usual energy, so this collage is neater than some I made when I was feeling sick.

CD 67: In a sense, I had graduated too.

CD 68: The back cover of the altered book shows the progression of my healing, symbolized by the growth of my hair, from my mossy head to myself now.

I found the altered book to be the perfect vehicle for me to tell my can-cer story. A history of this art form, which is both relatively new and quite old, is recounted in the Appendix.

Following the Altered Book on the CD are additional pictures in color that appear in black and white in the text, designated by their corre-sponding figure numbers.

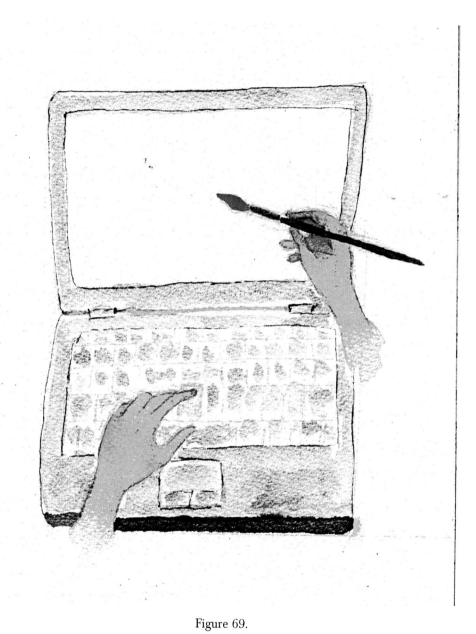

Figure 69.

6

WRITING AND MAKING ART

Throughout the creation of this work, I have been aware that the processes of writing and making art differ for me, both in the nature of the experiences and in their results. Together, however, I believe that each has enhanced the expressive qualities of the other. Although I have certainly been aware of some of these differences in the past, the focus of telling my story of my life with cancer in these two modalities has highlighted the different potentials of each.

WRITING

My written journal is a small dark-blue leather loose-leaf notebook. The jagged scrawl of my script reflects how sick I was feeling from day to day. Eventually, my computer took over for the discussions after treatment ended.

During treatment, however, there were many days I had to force myself to open my journal and write. When I was feeling especially sick, I recorded the day's events and that was it. I tried to include my reactions to what was happening to me, but sometimes I was just too exhausted or nauseous or depressed. During the time I was keeping the journal, I never read over what I had written. I didn't want to look at it. It was too painful. At some later date, I typed the journal pages onto the computer. I hated the tedium of typing the written notes that flung me back into the experience of my cancer treatment. When it ended after six months, I stopped writing my daily experiences. I was finished. It was a relief to be released in more ways than one: released from the chemo and the sickness and fatigue it brought on and re-

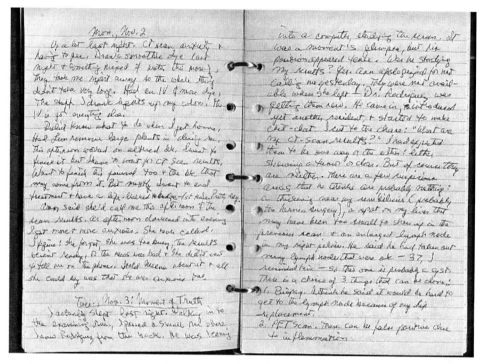

Figure 70. My journal.

leased from writing every day's events, including what sometimes felt like trivia.

At other times during the whole process, however, I wrote commentaries and elaborated on my thoughts. These interrupted the chronicling of events. I liked writing these portions. I liked reflecting. I liked finding metaphors. I liked going to the heart of what was happening to me.

Once both treatment and my journal had ended, however, I realized that I was still contending with my cancer and that I had much more to say. Although I was feeling well and longed to return to my prior life, that was not possible. Cancer does not end with the completion of treatment and the return to feeling well. It became important to me to record the aftermath of cancer treatment, especially my great anxiety at some of my medical checkups and my efforts to resurrect my life. Rather than scrawling in a notebook, I wrote the section on "Surviving" that follows the daily journal mostly on my computer. In contrast with some of the journaling that I had to force myself to write, I enjoyed thinking on my computer in this way. I liked writing only when I had something to say, rather than feeling bound to chronicle all I was experiencing.

Now, however, many months later, I am grateful that I did chronicle the events that were happening to me because I am beginning to forget much of what I went through during treatment. Although I had never intended my writing to serve as a record of this whole experience, it has done just that. I can now look at what I have written with less pain and with gratitude for the memory that the written word provides. I can remember the feelings and plumb them more deeply. This is the writing I like to do.

What else do I get from writing besides a record? I bring coherence to the kaleidoscope of my experience. I tell my story. In some way, difficult to explain, I become more of who I am. I think this kind of individuation is important for those living in the shadow of cancer's sickness and fatigue, its enforced dependency, unceasing dread, and what may be harsh, debilitating, and sometimes humiliating treatment. As I said in the Introduction, it is easy to become your cancer. It can suck out all other life you have, but creative self-expression can affirm your own special personhood, what in you is strong and unique. Cancer can seem like a dark cave into which you have fallen that separates you from others and even from yourself, the person you knew before the onslaught of the disease. Tangible self-expression can form a bridge to others to tell them what it is like for you to live in Cancer Land. In writing, I have asserted that I am more than a cancer victim, a recognition that was and still is important to me. I see myself as the unique individual I have always been but now even more so for having withstood cancer and its torture treatment in my own way.

For anyone afflicted with cancer, reaction to this illness is complex. There is a whirlwind of emotions. Most of us have gone to hell and back. We may have discovered who our friends are and who loves us. We may have sorted out what is important in our lives. For me, writing it all down was imprinting the experience, like an intaglio, in my consciousness. This is who I am. This is how I have borne this hardship. Cancer changes you. It has tempered me to become the person I am now. My writing is the log of this treacherous journey.

MAKING ART

Making art had a totally different effect on me. When I could do nothing else, write or read, take a walk or converse with a friend, I could make art. There were times I felt so awful that it was too much to get up from the table to reach the shelf for the kind of glue I needed for a collage or for a particular color of paper, so I just used what I had at hand on the table. The result was sometimes sloppy. Nevertheless, I was completely absorbed.

How to portray chemo brain, chemo stomach, peripheral neuropathy? I found ways. I glued my shed hair to pages of the altered book. The radiation treatment was so barbaric that I drew it more abstractly, shying away from its graphic horrors. Hours would pass without my noticing, and the day would be gone. I'd end up exhausted but strangely satisfied.

How can I explain the transcendence of making art? I would sit at the table in my office/studio with my supplies around me—paint, brushes, papers, glue, ribbons, magazine images, scissors, water, paper towels—some of it overflowing onto chairs, but all of it within reach. I'd have an idea—maybe gluing my lost hair into the book—and I would gather up what I would need. I'd assemble, draw, paint, cut, glue. My mind would be with my materials, formulating the image I wanted to create. This kind of intense focus is all encompassing, upstaging the world of nausea, fatigue, and constant dread. Paradoxically, even though the subject of my art was often the ravages of my treatment, the making of it lifted me out of it. When I had finished a piece, I had the satisfaction of looking at my own creation and finding it aptly expressive. Crude as many of these pictures were, they gave me pleasure even as they depicted pain.

I am an art therapist. My working life has been built upon the premise that making art can help people in many different ways. My patients and clients, and even my students, have shown me how this happens, but the art of my clients and patients develops with my encouragement, usually in my presence. The art therapist is an essential component of the art therapy equation. Sometimes I am a silent witness. At other times, I offer encouragement or react with questions to help in exploring the art and the self. There are times when I provide a focus or an art method, introducing new projects that might be stimulating. It is a shared journey, especially in finding meaning in the art. My cancer art did not include the presence and support of an art therapist. I believe the whole enterprise would have been very different if I had been working as an art therapy patient. How the art would have turned out had I been in therapy, I cannot say.

Unlike many of my clients and patients, I was accustomed to making art so I needed no encouragement. Similar to much of their art, one of the necessary aspects of my cancer art was that it had to be art that could be made relatively easily and quickly. Most of the time I was working on it, I felt too sick for the extended work necessary for more ambitious projects. Because I was alone in expressing and exploring myself, I had no expectation that anyone else would see my art. Occasionally, Neena came in and asked to see what I was making, and I did take the book in its initial stage to the Altered Book Workshop's second session, but that was it. When the book was almost completed, I showed it to a few friends, but clearly, I was making it only for me. It became a gift to myself, both in creating it and in the finished product. It was a part of cancer that felt good.

There have been other times in my life when making art helped me to deal with both physical disability, such as recovery from hip replacement surgery, and emotional turmoil, such as grief from the death of my father. I believe my cancer art, however, has been more extensive than any other single focus my art has had. It did not cure me of cancer. It did not alleviate the discomfort, it did not cheer me up, but it asserted in me what is strong, powerful, and creative. The artwork did not transform my cancer–that was not possible–but it did make some part of the experience worthwhile for me. That is the transcendent quality of creativity.

COMPARING WRITING AND MAKING ART

Just as the processes of writing and making art have been different for me, the results are also different. We are a verbal society. Telling is how we communicate. In writing, I could describe what happened and how I felt about it. I could write down what the doctor said and my reaction to his words. I could read my journal and be reminded of Neena arranging her calendar to drive me wherever I needed to go or of how unready I felt to be kicked out of the hospital three days after my surgery. Writing is literally literal.

Although we speak to one another in words, images surround us. What we see and how we see influence us, perhaps more than we know. As I tell my art therapy students, we think in images as well as in words, but we had images way before we knew the meaning of words. We could recognize our mothers before we had a name for her. Images are a more primitive source of knowing our world.

In many instances, the art I created was more metaphoric than my written journal was. The altered book has a black hole burrowed through its pages. That was my life—a black hole into which everything was sucked. Somewhat abstract or surreal images often best expressed how I felt, such as the pictures of chemo stomach, chemo brain, and neuropathy. The last pages are "After." While I was living in the black hole, I was making pictures of what I wanted to do when I got out of it: images of travel to exotic places, going to the theater and being out of doors, photos of the people I love, my children and grandchildren who live far away, with whom I wanted to spend time. It was important to be able to visualize a future free of misery. Creating pictures of what I wanted to do made these possibilities come to life for me.

The sequencing of events differed in the order in which I wrote about them and in which I depicted them in art. Clearly, the written portion is much more systematic than the altered book is. I tried to write every day during the six months of my treatment. Both during and afterward, I also wrote on subjects of particular interest to me and certain nodal experiences that occurred after completion of treatment. Although the artwork also had a chronicling nature and appears in the book in a temporal sequence, it was not created in that way. Whereas in writing I was recounting experiences and reactions soon after they occurred, in making art, the sequence of events was often shuffled. For example, my first art piece was a picture of death. In needing to make pictures of life after treatment while I was undergoing the worst of it, I was working on the ending of the book before the beginning and middle. In a way, the writing about events was more timely. The art making was more retrospective.

Now that I have finished both, I find interesting what I have included and what I have omitted in each part. It is only now in looking back that I am aware of omissions. I am not sure what to make of them. There are many more omissions in the artwork than in the writing, probably due to the chronicling process of my journal. It never occurred to me, for example, to make art about my many trips to the Botanic Gardens, although I certainly found them very nurturing. I entered them in my written journal, but I suppose there was nothing about them that called forth an image I wanted to create, despite their beauty. The art was certainly less of a record than the writing was.

Neena brought my attention to an omission in the writing that surprised her. Only in the last stages of completing this work have I given her the manuscript to peruse. She was surprised that I had omitted the couple therapy that had been so important to her. I hadn't thought to include it. It began after my daily chronicling, but perhaps more significant, it may not have been as meaningful to me as it was to her. (I have now included it, however, because I do believe it was useful.)

If there is any sort of explanation I can come up with for omissions in the artwork, I believe it centers on my inner experience. Although the altered book has pages about other people, my family and friends, caregivers, and so on, for the most part the focus is on what was happening to me, often representations of physical and emotional experiences, such as surgery, chemotherapy and its side effects, radiation, and wishes for the future. The symbolic, metaphoric nature of art lends itself more to this sort of expression than just to the literal, whereas words capture happenings more readily. For example, the obsessing about living arrangements was not so close to my inner experience for me ever to consider making art about it, even though I used my writing to process my thoughts about what I wanted to do. I wrote also about my pervasive digestive problems because they were such a significant aspect of my discomfort, even though I found sharing this experience with others embarrassing. It never occurred to me to make art about it.

An altered book by its structure imposes a space limit, whereas writing can go on and on. When I reached the altered book's last page and back cover, I had to finish. As a result, the ending is somewhat arbitrary. Although I changed the ending from Thanksgiving to graduation and added the progression of my hair growth on the back cover, after that, I was totally out of pages. None of the material in the "Surviving" section of the written journal appears in the altered book, except for the last page and back cover, because the art book was essentially completed right after the CAT scan that signaled the end of my treatment. I did make additional pictures about my cancer experience after completing the altered book, however, such as the crab I drew in my Northwestern class and the painting of bone marrow, both included here.

In the written journal, I found myself writing on and on. In a way, cancer has no ending, so I had to pick an arbitrary point at which to stop. In actuality, I had planned to end the journal earlier than I did, but then I was faced with new, unexpected challenges that I wanted to include. Of course, in both media it would be possible to plan in advance an ending and all that would lead up to it, but that was not the kind of expressive outlet I needed. I was tracking my life with cancer as I was living it.

GOING PUBLIC

As I have said, I did not write my cancer journal in order to publish it. I was writing for myself alone. As I was writing my journal, I did not show it to anyone, not even to my partner Neena. Looking at art is different from reading, and I did show my altered book to Neena and a few friends. In a way, the images could be more distant than the words, so I felt less vulnerable about them. I could say very little and let the viewers take from looking at them what they would. They could flip through the pictures quickly; they did not have to spend time with them. It was in combination with the written portions that I felt the images had their more significant impact.

I am a writer, however, and at some time in the progression of my journal days, I thought about publishing. I'm not sure when it was, but I think there were two major influences. The first was the OCWW's presentation by Patricia Lear on memoirs about major illnesses. That was an opportunity I was determined not to miss, even though I feared I would be too sick to attend because the date was two days after my last chemo treatment. I did become very sick from it and had to be hospitalized (chemo reactions are cumulative) but fortunately not until two days after the workshop. Like other writers who speak at OCWW meetings, Patricia offered to critique fifteen pages of related manuscripts. She would accept the first ten submitted. Although, looking back, I realize that it was unlikely she would receive that number from this group, at the time I thought this was an opportunity I would not have again, so I rushed my submission of fifteen pages to her. I didn't even stop to think about whether I wanted others to see such personal ruminations, especially since I shied away from reading them myself. As is the custom, the speaker selects some submissions to read aloud anonymously to the group and discuss. Mine was chosen. My friend Sue, who is an actor, volunteered to read it aloud and did so with much emotion. The audience seemed very moved. I was encouraged. When Patricia asked if the author wanted to identify himself/ herself, I stood. This was a sort of "coming out" for me. I considered publication.

After the OCWW experience, I decided to put the words and images together for a presentation to my Portia group. This would be more of a test of others' reactions to the whole work. Portia meets once a month and one of us presents her work, usually a work in progress. Over the years, I have presented my work a number of times, often a chapter from a book I was writing, one time a sort of retrospective of my art, and once even an experiential art-making workshop in which I led the others in some art exercises. This time, I read portions from my journal and showed the art that went with them. My presentation was too long, so periodically I asked if I should stop. No, they said. This group of bright, creative women was enrapt, not just interested as they had been at my other presentations. They told me the work was "inspirational." That did it for me. I contacted a publisher.

Since then, I have presented the altered book at an art show at the Cancer Wellness Center and some of the artwork to the Illinois Art Therapy Association, to art therapy students at The Art Institute of Chicago, and more recently at the AATA Annual Conference, from which they made an online distance learning course, but I felt particularly vulnerable about showing such personal expressions of my own artwork to my peers at the conference. My presentation played to a packed house, and the response was wonderfully positive, with members of the audience thanking me profusely. For the remaining days of the conference, people stopped me in the halls to tell me they had had cancer or a parent had, and for the first time they understood what their parent had gone through.

Despite these positive responses, I am still unsure about reactions from others to this book. During treatment, when I read other illness memoirs, mostly cancer experiences, I suffered as I did so. For the most part, they frightened me, particularly as I read about recurrences and relapses, harsher medicines, and increased helplessness. I was glad for the authors who lived to tell their stories, despite their ghastly experiences with both the illness and its sledge-hammer treatment. Not all of them survived their cancers.

There are problems in publishing a fully honest memoir of illness. Some aspects of it are downright disgusting. I ask myself, do people really want to know the details of the unrelenting digestive problems surgery and chemo imposed upon me. If I want to give a full and honest picture of my existence at this time, however, I have to talk about the attention my disrupted gut claimed, the pain and malaise it caused. An even greater problem has been writing about other people who in some way failed me. In a few instances, I have changed identifying details. Fortunately, there were not many of these people and far more who were either very helpful or loving or both.

I consider much of the writing and the artwork raw. These are mostly spontaneous outpourings, not perfected and refined writings or art forms. Currently, I have in mind a large, complex painting I want to create of my entire cancer experience, a sort of synthesis of the many art pieces I made while I was undergoing treatment. I will probably paint it in oils or acrylics, and it will be a more thought-out synthesis of my cancer experience than the spontaneous images presented here. This might be my next project.

I suppose a reason I have wanted to publish this work has been to get some benefits out of what is otherwise mostly agonizing. So what is the good that can come from publishing this book? If you think money, forget it, nor do I expect fame. The understanding that can come from others, however, is precious. I would like that very much. If a recounting of my experience can be of any help at all to just one person with a deadly disease or to anyone caring for a cancer patient, writing this would be more than worth it. There may be those who find this book hard to read, as I did in reading the work of others. I can understand those who would rather not read the details of living with cancer, although I would hope that my present state of feeling well could be encouraging to them. I hope too that those who care for cancer patients will read this work, as well as other cancer memoirs. The more they can know of our experience, the more sensitive they can become in treating us.

Then there is just wanting to tell my story, wanting to express my personhood. I must admit that having people interested in reading and viewing my story is immensely affirming to me as a person and of my life. Thank you for reading.

As I write my last journal entries and digitize the artwork for publication, I recognize that this project has been more than creative expression to help me through the painful parts of my cancer treatment. It has served as a lens for reflection on my cancer experience and the year following treatment, forming a powerful synthesis for me. In completing this work for now, although in a way it is still unfinished with more to come, I can recognize how much it has meant to me to be working on an ongoing project. Building this book, creating something tangible from wisps of experience, has been immeasurably powerful in pulling me through the torments and terrors of cancer. When cancer's crab grabs you in the clutch of its claws, all other life can be squeezed out of you. As I have said, you can become your cancer. It is life sucking. For me, writing and painting and eventually putting together this book expressed that healthy part of myself that can be productive, even when besieged with disease and fear.

The therapist in me is tempted to urge others suffering with illness to engage in creative enterprises, but I don't want to proselytize. My efforts are only an example. Each of us must choose our own way.

I have often thought that words and images combined forge a dynamic power of expression. For me, they have helped me heal. They have helped me survive.

Appendix

HISTORY OF ALTERED BOOKS

The first people known to alter manuscripts were Italian monks during the eleventh century, who created new texts and illustrations, called palimpsest, by scraping the ink from earlier vellum manuscripts to recycle the valuable paper to be used again. In later centuries, altered books emerged as grangerism, a Victorian art form of illustrating books by gluing in engravings from other books. Making scrapbooks by pasting pictures and mementos onto the printed pages of old books was also a popular pastime from the late 1800s through the early 1900s (Maurer-Mathison, 2008).

Modern altered books began by accident in 1959 when Brion Gysin, an American painter and poet, was mounting drawings and cut through the *New York Herald Tribune* that had been placed behind his mounting boards. He found that the resulting strips of type from unrelated articles could be arranged to create new meanings. He began fashioning new narratives in this way with his friend, writer William Burroughs. They named their new process "Cut-up," and in addition to cutting pages, they scratched out words so that the changed juxtapositions established new meanings.

British artist Tom Phillips is credited with beginning the contemporary altered book movement. In 1965, he read a Burroughs interview and began experimenting with the cut-up process, which he called "column edge poems." Wanting to expand on the idea, he searched for an inexpensive book that would offer rich possibilities. He bought a used Victorian novel, *A Human Document* by W.H. Mallock, for three pence and began experimenting with altering it, working on the book for more than fifteen years. First, he marked out certain words to change the meaning of the text, and later began using collage and decoupage techniques and painting the book's pages with watercolor and gouache. He referred to the project as a "treated book." The finished product contains not only art, but also a novel, created entirely from the altered text of the original story. Phillips derived the title by folding the title page of the original so that *A Human Document* was transformed into *A Humument* (Phillips, 2008). This new work was first published in 1983. Images of *A Humument* can be viewed online.

A nonprofit organization, the International Society of Altered Book Artists (ISABA), was established to promote book altering as an art form (see www.alteredbookartistscom). The ISABA sponsors exhibitions and educational events. In the 1980s and 1990s, degree programs in book arts were developed, further establishing the book arts genre as fine art.

Other book-related art forms have developed as well, such as book sculpture, in which books may be shaped into new forms. For example, reliquaries and jewelry have been made from book pages, or an original form may be created with the characteristics of a book, such as pages or a booklike binding. Pop-up books, long popular in the children's book market, have entered the adult market, as well, in imaginative works, such as those by Nick Bantock. Some of his books are correspondences with envelopes and postcards inside, all decorated with his artwork (1991).

REFERENCES

Bantock, N. (1991). *Griffin & Sabine.* San Francisco: Chronicle Books.

Block, K. (2009). *Life over cancer.* New York: Bantam Books.

Butler, S., & Rosenblum, B. (1991). *Cancer in two voices.* San Francisco: Spinsters Book Co.

Cousins, N. (1970). *Anatomy of an illness.* New York: W. W. Norton.

Didion, J. (2005). *The year of magical thinking.* New York: Alfred A. Knopf.

French, M. (1998). *A season in hell: A memoir.* New York: Alfred Knopf.

Grealy, L. (1994). *Autobiography of a face.* Boston: Houghton Mifflin.

Host, C. (2009). *Between me and the river.* Don Mills, Ontario, Canada: Harlequin.

Jarvis, D. (2007). *It's not about the hair.* Seattle: Sasquatch Books.

Larkin, P. (2003). *Collected poems.* New York: Farrar, Straus & Giroux.

Lorde, A. (1980). *The cancer journals.* San Francisco: Aunt Lute Books.

Maurer-Mathison, D. (2008). *Collage, altered art and assemblage: Creating unique images and objects.* New York: Watson-Guptill.

Mukherjee, S. (2010). *The emperor of all maladies.* New York: Scribner.

Phillips, Tom, R. A. Introduction to a Humument. Available: http://www.humument.com/intro.html

Radner, G. (1989). *It's always something.* New York: Simon & Schuster.

Rich, K. R. (2000). *The red devil.* New York: Three Rivers Press.

Sigler, H. (1999). *Hollis Sigler's breast cancer journal.* New York: Hudson Hills Press.

Skloot, R. (2010). *The immortal life of Henrietta Lacks.* New York: Crown Publishing Division of Random House.

Taylor, J. B. (2006). *My stroke of insight.* New York: The Penguin Group.

Wadeson, H. (1980). *Art psychotherapy.* New York: John Wiley.

Wadeson, H. (2010). *Art psychotherapy* (2nd edition). Hoboken, NJ: John Wiley.

Wisenberg, S. L. (2009). *The adventures of cancer bitch.* Iowa City: The University of Iowa Press.

ABOUT THE CD-ROM

System Requirements

- A computer with a processor running at 120 Mhz or faster
- At least 32 MB of total RAM installed on your computer; for best performance, we recommend at least 64 MB
- A CD-Rom drive

Using the CD with Windows

To install the items from the CD to your hard drive, follow these steps:

1. Insert the CD into your computer's CD drive.
2. The CD interface will appear. The interface provides a simple point-and-click way to explore the contents of the CD.

Using the CD with Mac OS

To open the items on the CD, follow these steps:

1. Open the folder titled "For Mac OS"
2. It contains color images that are mentioned on pages 179-191 in the text, designated by their corresponding figure numbers.

Customer Care

If you have trouble with the CD, please call the support line at (800) 258-8980. Outside the United States, call (217) 789-8980. We will provide technical support only for installation and other general quality control items. For technical support on the applications themselves, consult the program's vendor or author.